One Week with us Can [...] Life

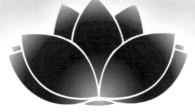

Ashland Brain Harmony

Experience Life Changing Benefits at Ashland Brain Harmony

- **Greatly Improve Sleep**
- **Increase Focus and Attention**
- **Experience More Happiness and Joy**
- **Enhance Spiritual Awareness**
- **Deepen Meditation**
- **Alleviate Symptoms of ADD, PTSD, Depression and Anxiety**
- **Increase Learning and Cognitive Abilities**
- **Decrease Addictive Behavior**
- **Enhance Sports Performance**

We work with Children, Adults, Seniors and Veterans

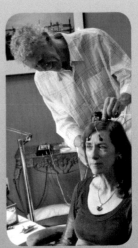

"I have had a life-long problem with insomnia and had Brainwave Optimization to help with that. Since finishing the training my sleep has been deeper and more restful. In addition, my mind is sharper with fewer extraneous thoughts and I am more able to focus for extended periods of time.

I highly recommend the Brainwave Optimization sessions to anyone. The training far exceeded my expectations."

~ Max Goler, Ashland, OR.

AshlandBrainHarmony.com
541-482-1542 • 180 Lithia Way

ADVANCE ACCLAIM FOR *LIMITLESS YOU*

I have fought my whole life to try to figure out what the heck was so different (and wrong) with me. I have always believed that I would find the answers to my many questions by listening to others (whom I always FELT were smarter than me) and that by doing what they said, I would find myself. So I tried EVERYTHING! After 43 years I had begun to lose faith in the process. I was beginning to make arrangements to settle for the truth that I was just going to have to accept the fact that I could not and would not ever be able to change. My experience at Brain State Technologies has re-established my faith in the healing process. For the very first time in my life I am keenly aware of what balance and harmony feels like. Brain training has given me a sense of hope again. I have begun a new journey to self-discovery and I can feel myself changing and making healthier choices for myself. If I can feel/believe like this, anyone can. I am living proof that if you show up and wait for God to walk through the room, your miracle can and will happen.

Wynonna Judd
Nashville, TN

In a world on the verge of a major shift in science and medical practice, the research performed by Lee Gerdes and his colleagues has established an innovative and more holistic approach to neurophysiology and behavioral disorders as a whole. This model merges neuroscience, quantum physics, and psychology to create a powerful technology that, I believe, will help heal humankind.

Riccardo Cassiani-Ingoni
PhD in Neurophysiology
University of Rome, Italy

Limitless You is a book about hope, choices, and boundless human potential. Lee Gerdes has tackled the vast complex territory of the human brain, and has given us a highly readable, informative, and inspiring book about how people can change the dysfunctional patterns that have been limiting their lives. In a clear and systematic style, Lee explains how our feelings, thoughts, and behaviors are often determined by patterns that are hard-wired into our brain, leaving us helpless to change. As a psychologist who has worked with people seeking freedom from their suffering for the past twenty-five years, I have been frustrated by the limitations of talk-therapy. With the introduction of revolutionary brain training technology, Lee Gerdes powerfully demonstrates how we can learn to transform the old neural patterns and achieve a brain that is functioning in balance and harmony with itself. As the stories in the book so beautifully illustrate, when the brain is in balance, everything else just works better. This book is essential to anyone who is interested in moving beyond human limitations to living life at the highest potential. As life in the twenty-first century becomes more challenging, I predict that brain training will become a household term and that *Limitless You* will become one of the most important books of our time.

Dr. Susan Simpson
Psychologist and Director of Waves of Potential
Vancouver, BC

As an integrative medical doctor, I'm always looking for faster, cheaper, and more effective ways to solve patient problems. The day I learned what brain training could offer, I scheduled an appointment. Within a week, I noticed a major improvement in my mood, energy, focus, ability to organize my thoughts, and balance. Of course, my tennis game also improved! Since that time, I've referred patients for brain training with depression, anxiety, and post-traumatic stress disorder. Their comments universally: "It changed my life." I think Lee Gerdes is an absolute genius to have advanced this technology to this level. Read the book. But more important, experience the benefits.

Linda Wright, MD
Board Certified Internal Medicine
Scottsdale, AZ

In my search for a complimentary method that would help my clients who were dealing with obsessive thoughts and/or behaviors, I found Brain State Technologies three years ago. Since then, I have discovered the myriad of enhancements that BST can offer, and have referred numerous people of varying ages (7-60), continually being impressed by their changes and achievements. I believe any practitioner, in any modality, would find that brain training offers a seamless and effective compliment to anyone's work in helping people live a happier and healthier life. *Limitless You* takes the reader step by step through an understanding of how the brain affects our behavior, how brain training works, and the kind of changes people are experiencing in their lives—changes similar to which I've observed in my clients and personally experienced.

Kim M. Evans
President, Life Changing Solutions and Certified Rubenfeld Synergist
Scottsdale, AZ

Through his understanding of brain patterns, quantum physics, mathematics, and highly advanced computer technology, Lee Gerdes, in his book *Limitless You*, gives us great insight into how adversely a trauma can affect the brain and further explains how Brain State Technologies was able to develop a remarkably effortless yet extraordinarily successful "brain training" method that allows the brain to rebalance and harmonize after a trauma has been imprinted. Not only does this new technology give us a glimpse into the future, it gives us great hope that the future is NOW.

Trudy Peters
Co-author of Owen's Choice *and* Andre's Choice

Lee Gerdes provides us with a powerful and compelling book written from his direct experience as a brain trainer. Liberally peppered with individual stories, Gerdes' book demonstrates how radically people's lives have changed for the better with little effort on their part. You will want to try this method for yourself, whether you have serious problems or just want to live more comfortably in your skin.

Duane Groce, MS
Author, The Inner Switchboard

LIMITLESS YOU

LIMITLESS YOU

The INFINITE POSSIBILITIES
of a
BALANCED BRAIN

Lee Gerdes

Namaste Publishing
Vancouver, Canada

Library and Archives Canada Cataloguing in Publication

Gerdes, Lee, 1945–
   Limitless you : the infinite possibilities of a balanced brain / Lee Gerdes.

   Includes bibliographical references.
   ISBN 978-1-897238-41-7

   1. Brain. 2. Mind and body. 3. Homeostasis. 4. Sound—Therapeutic use. 5. Mental healing. 6. Mental health. 7. Electroencephalography. 8. Self-actualization (Psychology). I. Title.

RC386.2.G47 2008   616.8   C2008-906289-2

Published by NAMASTE PUBLISHING
PO Box 62084
Vancouver, BC, Canada V6J 4A3
www.namastepublishing.com
namaste@telus.net

Distributed in North America by HAMPTON ROADS PUBLISHING COMPANY
Charlottesville, VA
hrpc@hrpub.com

Cover design by Amy King
Interior book design by Val Speidel
Printed and bound in Canada by Friesens

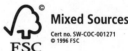

Mixed Sources
Cert no. SW-COC-001271
© 1996 FSC
FSC

All of the case histories referred to in this book are of actual people. However, while in the case of some, such as Justin, where the person's real name and circumstances have been preserved, the names and circumstances of others have been changed to protect the privacy of the individuals, their family members, and other significant personages in their stories.

To Peter Gerdes, who walked this walk with me;

to Brain State staff, who were asked to accept
a cut in pay and work more hours,
and did it because of the love they share
for the greater good;

to Brain State affiliates all over the planet,
who seek well-being for everyone they touch;

and mostly, for the approximately 10,000 people
around the world who have utilized brain training
in their search for well-being and to help
optimize their lives—you have honored us
by allowing us to be of assistance.

Contents

15

16

17

18

Acknowledgments

MANY THANKS to the dozens of doctors, scientists, psychotherapists, theologians, and neurofeedback providers who have helped me understand what this inner journey to optimize the brain is all about and who advised me how information processing is accomplished in quantum space.

I want to give heartfelt thanks to the efforts of Peter Gerdes, for his trust and for his years of dedicated work, which included working at times with limited tools and in adverse conditions. Also, to Laura (Gerdes) Osier, who trusted her dad to use his technology.

Brain training was born out of a need to solve my own problem. I want to thank all of those in the helping professions who sustained me for many years and thereby gave me an opportunity to discover a solution that worked best for me.

This book would not have been possible without Constance Kellough, President and Publisher of Namaste Publishing, who recognized the importance of the work, and David Robert Ord, Editorial Director for Namaste Publishing. Thank you for your thoughtful and heartfelt work, and for using the technology yourselves to ascertain its safety and efficacy.

Brain State Technologies™ has many individuals associated with its work who have been instrumental in bringing this technology to the world. Paul Hastings and Russ Loucks have worked with me for over ten years as dedicated and creative software developers whose brains are huge and whose hearts are just as big. Alexa Bolles was the first Brain State affiliate and is now Director of Sales and Marketing, using her skills to usher others into this world of helping people through this non-invasive technology. The many individuals who work for Brain State have shown up to work, care for clients, bring this technology to the world, and sustain it in excellence.

I acknowledge the ten percent of clients who were not sufficiently assisted by the technology, but worked to seek a better life for themselves and those around them. They taught me much along the way and helped us hone the efficacy of the technology as we developed new approaches to brain training.

Lastly, I acknowledge my ninety-eight-year-old mother, Josephine Margaret (Thies) Gerdes of Auburn, Nebraska, whose son listened sufficiently to know that we each have huge potential and that seeking this potential and finding its role for the well-being of all is key to a life well lived. She is my best friend, and I honor all that she believed was good by striving to help people and move them toward an optimized state for the greater good of the world.

Foreword

UNTIL RECENTLY, the dominant scientific belief was that our brain is a machine. In this view, if you injured a part of your brain, as in trauma, you lost that function. This is because the brain was seen as a fixed entity that's hardwired.

However, thanks to advances in neuroplasticity—the study of how the human brain can change itself—this concept no longer holds. We now know that our brain can rewire itself to attain its fullest capacity, including the regaining of higher mental functions.

At the heart of *Limitless You* is the author's conviction that we can train our brain to change our life. He sees a Brain Fitness Revolution on the horizon, which will bring balance to our lives simply by training an unbalanced brain to an optimum state. The book is a fascinating constellation of illustrations of human potential.

This revolutionary technology demonstrates that what is happening inside the brain is more significant in terms of the quality of our life than what comes to us from the external world. Lee Gerdes writes movingly about the ways in which this extremely innovative approach is being used to change brain wave energy and hence enrich people's lives.

Limitless You is an informative overview of how we can become more in tune with ourselves, experience spiritual healing, reduce post-traumatic stress disorder, relieve stress and anxiety, rid ourselves of addiction, become less impulsive, curb tendencies to anger and violence, and enhance the overall quality of our lives. Brain training is an especially ideal fit with more natural approaches to wellness.

The book demonstrates the scope and power of brain training by citing numerous examples of people who suffer from a whole spectrum of conditions in which the underlying defect is an unbalanced brain. When the brain returns to a state of balance and harmony, the individual is able to function optimally. Coming from a diverse educational background in math, physics, psychology, and theology, the author shares accounts of individuals who have already benefited from this innovative technology with sensitivity and compassion. He has succeeded in capturing not only the person's spiritual transformation, but also the physiological aspects of this transformation.

To me personally, the book is a remarkable and hopeful portrayal of the endless possibilities of the human brain to empower us to take charge of our lives. Balance your brain and you will lead a happier life.

Limitless You is all about listening to the sounds of your brain, body, and soul.

Vijendra Singh, PhD, Neuroscientist

Introduction

WE HAVE KNOWN for a long time that a connection exists between mind, body, and spirit, but now we can observe this connection. We can see it at work through technology, and more important, we can actually improve the way it functions.

The brain acts as the hub of the wheel of our life. The nervous system can be likened to the spokes of a wheel, while the body is the rim. When the hub is out of balance, everything else is affected. Instead of enjoying a relatively smooth and almost effortless ride through life, our days are often marked by drama and trauma.

This book introduces a modality known as Brain State Conditioning™, which is widely referred to as brain training and is oriented toward solving problems related to brain energy. Brain training isn't based on diagnosis and neither is it concerned with any symptoms a client may be suffering. Rather, its focus is on the degree of *balance* and *harmony* the brain experiences, plus the flexibility it demonstrates when it moves from being at rest to being activated. This is quite different from modalities that compare a person's brain with a normative database and then try to teach the individual to bring their brain functioning up to par with the average brain.

When we talk about *balance,* we are talking about how the brain's activity is balanced from one hemisphere of the brain to the other, and also how the different regions of the brain balance with each other between the front and back of the same side of the brain. Brain training facilitates brain balance. It's like loading a ship so that it's level on the ocean.

When we talk about *harmony,* we are referring to how energy patterns that vary from low to high exist together in the same region of the brain.

If you have ever driven an automobile with one or more tires out of balance, you know the shimmy and shake that an out-of-balance condition can produce. Well, it's no different in life when the brain has one or more of its regions out of balance. In such a condition, it simply isn't possible to live a life of excellence.

When the brain is balanced and in harmony, it can have a dramatic effect on both the mind and the body. For this reason, brain balance and harmony can be a helpful step to a state of well-being and optimum performance.

When the brain is balanced and in harmony, people involved in sports are much more likely to achieve optimum performance in terms of speed, strength, and so on. Writers, musicians, and artists achieve greater creativity and artistic expression. Individuals who feel stuck—who realize they aren't living up to their full potential but don't know how to let their true being out—often advance to gratifying business endeavors. Whatever a person's walk of life, they can gain clarity about their life's journey.

A Chance to Take Charge of Your Life

Brain training doesn't require *willpower*. Instead, it uses *brainpower*.

Our society is wedded to the idea that we all have free will and simply need to make good choices then stick to them. We have drunk so deeply of this philosophy that we don't realize how limited a person's ability to make good decisions is when their brain is in an unbalanced state. Individuals also tend to lack the willpower to engage in the difficult and often ongoing struggle it takes to change an entrenched pattern of behavior. For instance, countless people with the best of intentions tell themselves, "I'm going to stop smoking." They recognize quitting their habit would make a tremendous improvement in their life. But those who attempt this find it isn't easy, and many fail despite repeated efforts. For most of us, it requires more than willpower.

Using brainpower to change our lives takes the struggle out of it. It's all about achieving self-improvement from a place of deep calm. Our brain learns to function in a more wholistic way.

One client tells how she actually experienced the difference: "I thought education was about information; I thought discipline was about control; I thought procrastination was about willpower; and I thought stopping bad habits and behavior was supposed to be hard, and sustaining new behavior even harder. I was wrong. It isn't about willpower, it's about brainpower. I was at a crossroads. I was smoking and felt like the rat who couldn't learn. My daughter told me that, as an intelligent woman, I should be embarrassed to end up dying from a preventable disease. But I had tried everything and could not stop. It took me a few hours of training to stop smoking, but it took me nearly thirty-five years to find the technology that helped me stop."

A brain that's balanced and in harmony is in a state known as homeostasis. The term is derived from two Greek words, *homoios* meaning "same" and *stasis* meaning "stand." In a state of homeostasis, conditions stay the same. It's a state in which the brain functions on a level playing field, which enables it to respond to life's challenges in an optimal manner. When the brain is in homeostasis, thinking, feeling, performing, and the body's ability to repair itself all function at their best and self-regulate based on what they are called upon to do at any given moment.

Brain training is potentially a life-changing tool, serving as an adjunct to other modalities with the objective of helping these modalities achieve what they seek to accomplish by first bringing the person into a state of self-regulation. Also, when used as a non-invasive information-gathering tool, as a means of exposing causes and effects, brain training illuminates the path to how countless disorders might be corrected more quickly and more completely.

Brain training is a revolutionary way to break free from our limiting history. It allows retraining of the imbalances in the brain to help correct various disorders without negative side effects or invasive procedures.

Doctors are told, "First, do no harm," but unfortunately, many of the pharmaceuticals and procedures currently in use have devastating side effects for some. Brain training is a tool to help "do no harm." It isn't the only answer, but I believe it is part of the solution—a part that may be the missing link when it comes to ADHD, sleep issues, postmenopausal problems, depression, anxiety, pain management, addiction, and the quest for optimum performance.

Take addiction, which is often seen as difficult to change, but for brain training poses no greater challenge than any of the other dysfunctions many of us experience from day to day. After an addict does brain training to balance and harmonize their brain patterns, they are unlikely to desire their addiction. Their brain can be assessed and trained, often with stunning results. For example, in an efficacy trial with probationers in Yavapai County, Arizona, brain training made it possible for repeat offenders with long histories of addiction, including prolonged methamphetamine use, to begin a new life. Even though the trial participants remained in constant contact with other addicts, after the first year more than eighty-five percent remained substance free. After three years, of the participants surveyed, more than seventy-five percent were still substance free—an astounding accomplishment compared with conventional approaches.

The process is simple, and it works with other conditions and disorders with the same glaring simplicity.

How Brain Training Was Discovered

People who have trained their brain often want to know about my background. How did I come up with this simple yet powerful modality?

I wasn't a doctor or even a brain researcher; I was a computer geek. Most of my life revolved around computer science, though my background did include a degree in theology and extensive work in psychology as well as math and physics.

As Vice President of Solutions for Net Perceptions in Minneapolis, I was consulting and designing software along with developing algorithms for marketing. In essence, an algorithm is a formula, and the Net Perceptions algorithms linked similar products or concepts to individuals. Our first customer was Amazon.com, which licensed technology that notes the kind of books a person buys then suggests other books they might also enjoy. You've probably seen the recommendation, "If you liked … you may like …" Our original Net Perceptions algorithms are still widely used in today's marketplace.[1]

We were a successful company whose stock was climbing when web-based stocks suddenly fell dramatically in a general collapse of web-based businesses at that time. Such businesses were often greatly overvalued because people's expectations of what a web-based business could achieve were inflated. When it became clear that many of these businesses weren't going to be profitable, investors started pulling their money out, leading to widespread panic.

However, Net Perceptions had already proven successful, so our initial response during the crisis was to find still wider uses for our technology. I headed up a team that built a business-to-business application whereby we could assist, for example, an electrical store that stocked tens of thousands of parts to achieve a much more efficient turnover of its stock. When a contractor comes in to order parts, our algorithm figures out what parts they might have overlooked so they won't have to return for them at a later date. Through all of this, I was gaining increasing proficiency in software design, having worked in the software field since the sixties.

I was suffering from post-traumatic stress disorder. To try to alleviate this condition, I sought out one healing modality after another. Though I went through a raft of treatments in addition to extensive psychotherapy, such treatments were of only limited help. Though to some degree they alleviated my physical condition, they were unable to affect the edge I was on all the time. Anyone could press my buttons and evoke a lightening-fast response—a response out of proportion to what was appropriate, and a huge waste of emotional energy.

Alongside my fascination with computer software development, I had a deep interest in science, especially quantum mechanics. The development of brain training was, in a way, an accident. Among the more helpful therapies I had tried were biofeedback and neurofeedback. Suddenly, it occurred to me how the insights of quantum mechanics, teamed with highly sophisticated computer technology, could enable an individual to go so much further than was possible with either biofeedback or neurofeedback.

It was only when I tried training my own brain with the first technology and protocols I developed that I finally felt better. After benefitting from the technique for some weeks, I set it aside, never imagining it would someday help thousands of people.

My son began having problems during the usual rebellious stage of the teen years. Falling in with a tough crowd, he left school, experienced some difficulties with a girlfriend, and was rapidly going downhill toward a dysfunctional life. I believed he could benefit from the brain training I had used on myself, so I essentially bribed him to give it a try. I sent him a computer, amplifier, and electrodes. The effect was stunning. He cleaned up his life, returned to school, and immediately made the dean's list.

With my encouragement, my son then tried the technique on several other people, which made him not only my first real client but also my first trainer. It was his success, along with the success of his friends, that spurred us to make the training available to other people and led me to leave Net Perceptions. Now, thousands have found a way out of their self-limiting prisons by utilizing brain training. All it took was balancing their brainwave patterns.

From Simple to Sophisticated

Brain training began with a mobile office. I hauled a computer and electronics in the back of my car. Volunteers were trained in their home, and the data we collected relative to the brain's response was used to refine the algorithms.

I had properties in Montana, Minneapolis, and Florida. I sold these and emptied my 401K. It was enough to set up the equipment required; still, I had a high level of anxiety over whether I was going to run out of money. I recall telling myself, "The universe is going to have to take it from here."

I moved to Scottsdale, Arizona, and my son and I lived together in a rented home with a bedroom on each side of the house. We set up a third bedroom as a lab and used the family room for research. We couldn't afford to pay our first associate; she came to work with us gratis until we could begin to reward her for her effort.

I can't tell you exactly how brain training started to mushroom; it just did. It was all by word of mouth, as people saw the lives of others change. At first many came to us who didn't have the financial means. They came because nothing else had worked for them and hence they had nothing to lose.

A few months later we were busier than we could have ever imagined. We moved to an office space, then we relocated to an even larger facility, and finally we moved into our current 18,000 square foot facility, still located in Scottsdale.

When brain training began, the technology was rudimentary compared to what we use today. We had 160 gigabytes of data storage capacity at startup, whereas at the time of this writing we have 18 terabytes. For the first three years, brainwaves were sampled at a rate of 128 samples per second, each with 256 bins of information. Now, 256 samples are taken every second, each with over 65,000 bins of information. This yields a vastly increased quantity of data, making brain training even more effective. We continually refine the technique based on the data we receive from over 10,000 clients, which comes to us online every twenty-four hours from more than a hundred and thirty licensees in over fifteen countries. This daily influx of data continues to inform our brain training protocols.

In case you are wondering what a brain training protocol is exactly, it consists of information fed back to the brain based on data collected by electrodes placed tactically on various areas of a person's head. Each brain training protocol is individually designed, and can last anywhere from five minutes to thirty minutes. A training session consists of approximately five to seven protocols, lasting in all about an hour and forty-five minutes. A person can participate in two training sessions a day, with at least two hours in between sessions to allow the brain to rest from the reorganizing of itself it has been doing during the earlier session.

A Technological Boom

Brain activity is manifested in electromagnetic energy, which can be measured. This energy is measured through tiny detection devices placed on the head. These brain energy detection devices (Intellectrodes™) are sophisticated forms of electrodes that contain a computer chip capable of picking up the tiny current of the brain in an entirely noninvasive manner. The brainwaves detected are replicated in a variety of colorful waveforms on a computer screen. The underlying science is electroencephalography (EEG).

Technologically speaking, when we examine brain functioning, we are looking at energy measured in the range of ten-millionths of a volt. With such an infinitesimal quantity of energy powering the brain, you can imagine how little it takes to cause interference. Detecting brain energy accurately, without interference, is far more delicate even than attempting to thread a needle when you are shaking from the chills!

Brain training utilizes a specific type of electrode that includes computer chips designed to eliminate other electromagnetic energy that might result in interference in the signals being detected. This is sophisticated hardware, which is coupled with highly sophisticated software. In fact, the developers who designed this software for us previously worked on supercomputers and devised a program that could build a molecule based on the characteristics they wanted the molecule to possess. To come up with even a sketch of such a molecule took six scientists two years, but the computer was able to build it in only two weeks. At that time, the supercomputer was the equivalent of running 100,000 desktop computers simultaneously. The computer technology used in brain training is facilitating advancements far beyond our understanding, but it isn't necessary for us to fully understand how it works in order to utilize this technology. In terms of building a brain training protocol in the future, the computer will make so many calculations from all the information it collects from the brain that we couldn't duplicate it in a lifetime of working with a desk calculator.

Intellectrodes™, coupled with other technological advances, are opening the way for us to see brain energy in 3,000 times the detail we could previously access. Imagine that we have gone from seeing the brain's energy with a ten-power microscope to seeing it with a 30,000-power microscope! Such detail will facilitate many new discoveries about how the brain works, allowing us to generate protocols that are more and more specific to the individual.

In other words, it's as if at one point we were looking at a mountain, then boulders on the mountain, then rocks that make up the boulders, and finally we are moving into seeing the energy that holds the rocks together. Or to use another analogy, it's the difference between looking at sugar cubes, granulated sugar, and powdered sugar. Consequently, if a woman with blue eyes and auburn hair were to come in for training, we might speculate from her brain map that she's really a blue-eyed blond. Think about this kind of breakdown of data in terms of pain management, for instance. Instead of having to address a wider region of the brain, we will be able to focus on the exact frequency in the brain where the discomfort is occurring.

As our technology advances, making it possible to look at smaller and smaller parts of brainwave frequencies, and as we collect more and more information in our data base to furnish us with an ongoing learning capability, it will become exponentially easier for us to achieve our potential as humans.

All of this has led me to wonder what we could do with the mind if our brain was truly its faithful servant. What would we become aware of if our brain was finely balanced?

Exploration of the brain is one of the cutting edge sciences on the planet today. The brain is the new frontier, and investigating this inner space is one of the most fascinating and rewarding adventures we will ever take. This book will give you some idea of the amazing achievements that are already possible with our present understanding of the brain.

1

Is It Really "All In Your Head?"

How does a seemingly calm teen who has never caused any trouble in his life get to the place where he decides to annihilate his fellow students and teachers?

Daniel, a seventeen-year-old, was stopped by the police on suspicion of drug possession. As they searched his car, they came across a notebook in which Daniel described his plans to carry out a massacre. The revelation was a shock to his parents, brother, and sister, who had emigrated from Eastern Europe to establish themselves as a respected and hardworking family on the eastern seaboard of the United States.

Daniel was angry because he felt that teachers and students at his school had shunned him. This feeling of isolation upset him so much that he began laying plans to eliminate them. Although many teens experience ostracism at times (school life can be cruel), most don't plan to retaliate with the massacre of their classmates and teachers. So why did Daniel's feelings of being left out lead him to plan something so incomprehensible?

The answer lies in the state of Daniel's brain. His neural network was unbalanced to the point that energy couldn't flow in the ways it does in a balanced brain. Consequently, Daniel lacked the ability to communicate fully and freely, which led others to avoid him. The frustration he experienced generated an intense need to break out of his isolation, to the point that he could actually contemplate harming those he believed were responsible for his isolation.

Fortunately for Daniel, the court system that processed his case was familiar with brain training and recognized it as a more viable way to address this young man's inability to function normally, believing it would afford him a better chance to return to a productive life in society. So instead of ordering that Daniel be committed to a psychiatric unit, the court recommended him for brain training.

No sooner did this teen begin training his brain than dramatic changes became apparent in his behavior. So great were the changes in their son that the father and mother signed up to train their brains as well.

Daniel's brain training sessions were followed by a residential substance abuse program, and the combination worked wonders. We'll talk even more about Daniel later in this chapter.

What a Brain Training Assessment Can Reveal

Brain training begins with an assessment of the individual's brain patterns. Performing a brain assessment is a straightforward process that involves no more than connecting one end of a set of electrodes to a computer, then placing the other end on the individual's head in a variety of different locations in order to detect the energy patterns of the brain.

The brain has a variety of lobes. A lobe is a region or neighborhood of the brain—much like a city might have a downtown shopping center, a business section, an industrial park, and residential suburbs. Just as each section of the city serves a different purpose, so do the lobes of the brain. Observing the activity in different lobes of the brain in an assessment procedure that lasts only forty-five minutes yields a wealth of information not only about the person's present brain state, but also about how past experiences may have contributed to this state, and hence to why people behave in self-destructive ways. Consider how many individuals addicted to alcohol or drugs lead directionless lives, oblivious of their potential. Why would anyone waste their life in this way? It's even more bewildering when someone who appears quite normal carries out a heinous act such as murder or a mass shooting. However, when the brain is assessed, the imbalance that led to such a heinous act is easy to see.

When Daniel's brain was assessed, it appeared he had experienced a severe trauma early in life. In fact, it seemed clear this trauma had occurred close to the time of his birth. But when the trainer asked his mother whether there had been any kind of difficulty during her son's birth, she responded, "No. The birth went smoothly."

"Well, I guess we can't be right all the time," the trainer commented. "Still, your son's brain assessment indicates a probability that his parasympathetic nervous system was strongly activated from an extremely early age, most likely before birth."

The sympathetic and the parasympathetic nervous systems together make up the autonomic nervous system. This system regulates the internal functions of the body, including heart rate, breathing, digestion, saliva, perspiration, size of the pupils, and sexual arousal. Much of what it does is automatic. For this reason, a person suffering from a head injury or stroke, who is in a vegetative state, is often still able to breathe and digest food. In a conscious individual, some functions of the autonomic nervous system can be controlled to a certain extent, breathing being a prime example.

The autonomic nervous system attempts to maintain a state of homeostasis in the body. The body employs a cascade of molecular mechanisms, including hormones and other chemical messengers, to regulate itself. For instance, if we step out of a cool house into a hot summer's sun, the body immediately begins perspiring in an attempt to cool itself, as it seeks to maintain the critical internal operating temperature that supports life. Similarly, when we eat a sugary dessert, the body signals the pancreas to release the hormone insulin in order to regulate our blood sugar level.

The sympathetic and parasympathetic nervous systems serve two different but complementary functions. Together, they work like an air pump. The pump stroke that forces air into the tire under pressure is the sympathetic system, whereas the pump stroke that opens the input valve to take in more air to pressurize the tire is the parasympathetic system.

There's an easy way to tell whether you are experiencing sympathetic or parasympathetic dominance. If you are driving down the street and a car runs a stop sign, nearly crashing into you, you are likely to find yourself shaking following the near impact, regardless of which system is dominant. But herein lies the difference. When you are experiencing sympathetic dominance, your initial thoughts are likely to be, "You idiot! You could have killed me." Or you might think, "Oh, God, was I going too fast?" or, "Did I have the right-of-way?" In other words, whether you place the blame on the other driver, or on yourself, you are likely to blame someone. However, if the parasympathetic system is dominant, there is a likelihood you will simply tremor, be unable to speak or think clearly for a few minutes, and require time to return to an awareness of your body so you can resume the task of driving to your destination.

Another way to understand whether you have a tendency to be sympathetic or parasympathetic dominant is to consider what you do when there is a confrontation or argument. If your first inclination is either to run or to fight, then it's likely you are sympathetic dominant. If however your inclination is to freeze—to not know what to say, and only later wish you had said a particular thing—then you are likely parasympathetic dominant.

Daniel's brain was parasympathetic dominant. But if his mother was correct and he hadn't suffered a trauma early in life, then there appeared to be no explanation for why his brain manifested such an imbalance.

The case presented a puzzle. How did Daniel's brain become so unbalanced if there had been no trauma or other external interference? Was it the result of a genetic flaw, or could it simply be a random occurrence? The mother had an easy delivery. She was in a loving relationship with the father. In fact, she insisted, "We have a great family." She also described her son as a "good baby." What, then, accounted for the huge imbalance in this "good baby's" teen brain? Why did he want to generate carnage at his school?

Brain science isn't a pure science yet. Although the indication of trauma as the source of a brain imbalance is accurate a high percentage of the time, it isn't a hundred percent accurate. Still, it seemed in this case that a key piece of the puzzle was missing.

Despite not knowing the cause of the imbalance, Daniel's brain assessment indicated there was a high likelihood the imbalance could be corrected, and ultimately this is the focus of brain training. It isn't necessary for people to know why they have a brain imbalance. In fact, in one sense the cause is irrelevant. The trainer simply identifies the imbalance then helps the person bring their brain back into balance.

It was during a later conversation with Daniel's mother that she related, "By the way, when I was eight months pregnant, I went to a picnic where I ate an excessive quantity of rich food that gave me indigestion. Thinking I was having labor pains, they took me to the hospital. The hospital also concluded I was having labor pains, so they began to induce me. But we had all calculated the wrong date, and as the induction proceeded, this became apparent. The ultrasound showed that, rather than preparing to be born, my baby had curled up into a ball and moved to the back of the womb. It was then that the hospital realized they had induced me a month early. They stopped the labor and gave me medication for my upset stomach. Could this have been the cause of our son's brain imbalance?"

There are numerous stories like this one. People simply don't realize how many things have happened in their life that were perceived by their brain as a threat, and how dramatically this can affect the brain's flow of energy. They are also unaware that these events are often responsible for the unhelpful brain patterns that manifest in dysfunctional behavior or physical pathologies later in life. Learning that it wasn't their fault the child they love went off the rails can be a tremendous relief to parents, who are often weighed down with terrible guilt.

Though Daniel's birth had been normal, inducement of the mother to deliver prematurely was an artificial assault on the gestation process, as a result of which his parasympathetic nervous system acted to protect him. Thank goodness it worked this way, because otherwise Daniel would have been born too early, a situation that would have carried with it a wide variety of risks and difficulties.

How the Brain Responds to a Threat

When, in an act of self-preservation, Daniel's brain created a pattern intended never to allow it to become so vulnerable again, it simultaneously worked against him. His parasympathetic nervous system, which protected him at the time of the attempted inducement, became stuck in a dominant mode.

One unhelpful brain pattern that can result when the parasympathetic nervous system becomes dominant is the state commonly referred to as a freeze response. When Daniel's brain caused him to ball up, he suffered an immense freeze response. His brain concluded, "Balling up saved my life," and it kept this as its dominant pattern. Stuck in maintaining a pattern that was absolutely essential at the time of the threat—a matter of survival—the brain didn't realize it could let go of this pattern without becoming vulnerable again.

Because this instinctive response enabled the brain to survive, it had all the proof it needed that its response was correct. If it could have done something different, such as run away from the scene or put up a fight, this may have become its pattern instead. In this example, Daniel couldn't run away and couldn't fight, so his brain did the only thing it could to make him safe. His brain caused him to freeze up, and this became his mode of self-preservation for the future.

As Daniel moved through life and encountered its many challenges, his unbalanced brain state caused him to respond in a manner that was subdued. Instead of actively engaging in life, he was largely frozen. Because he felt frozen, he became all but invisible. He was simply unable to respond in a fitting way. This freeze response is also the reason Daniel was perceived by others as a quiet, unassuming, good child. But inside, something quite different was developing.

When an individual's brain is extremely out of balance, the person is likely to behave in antisocial ways. For instance, when a person uses illegal substances, as Daniel was doing, it's often because their brain is out of balance. The substance is simply a way to self-medicate. Teens cutting themselves, pulling their hair out (trichotillomania), or becoming anorexic or bulimic also manifest an imbalance. To plan an act of violence is a manifestation of an extreme level of imbalance in the neural network, which is the vast array of pathways that channel the brain's energy. Planning the violence, though it was never carried out, was a way to excite the brain—to be in a fight-or-flight brain state rather than a freeze state.

Why the Teen Years Are So Challenging

When our children start down a path we know could lead them into serious trouble, we long to share our wisdom and steer them on a more wholesome course. But in our society, where young people are so heavily influenced by their peers, we sometimes feel shut out of their lives. It's a tremendous worry in millions of homes, and countless parents and guardians today are at their wits' end as to how they can help their troubled teens.

A recommendation one often hears is that parents should talk to their teens on a regular basis. If you've been a parent or caregiver, you know there comes a time when your teens may tune you out even as you are speaking. When you ask how their day was at school, all you get in response is, "Fine." Clearly, they don't want to communicate. When they're not out with their friends, they shut themselves off in their room, sending the clear message you are no longer welcome in their private life. This can be a challenging time for parents as well as their teenage children.

When young people begin behaving in dysfunctional ways, the parents usually express their concern. They feel that if they could just communicate with their kids—if they could only get them to listen—it would make such a difference. They attempt to steer the child in a healthy direction, but their advice falls on deaf ears because the teen's unbalanced brain is orchestrating their life. The usual teen response is, "Whatever!"

Suppose Daniel's mother had understood what happened a month before her son's birth and explained to him, "I was induced a month early, and when you balled up in the womb, they stopped the induction and you were born a month later." Would this knowledge have helped Daniel come to terms with the dangerous course his life was taking, enabling him to change his behavior? Possibly it would have made it easier for him to recognize his symptoms and to understand that the way he experienced the world was based on the imbalance in his brain. But it's unlikely this would have relieved his discomfort or alleviated his need to explode in rage in order to *feel* something—*anything*.

Many of us assume that if individuals are given the correct information, they will act on it. However, having the right information doesn't make everything all right. Most people who do terrible things know better, but they do them anyway. This is because they are driven by an imbalance that overrides their logic and their capacity to understand themselves as a viable part of the world in which they live.

It's not just rare events such as a threat to the fetus during gestation or a difficult situation during the actual birth that causes the brain to shift into an imbalance. As we shall see, all kinds of situations can trigger such a shift. Few of us grow to adulthood and retain a balanced neural network; and to the degree our brain is unbalanced, we will experience difficulties in life. The teen years, during which the stresses in life are exaggerated by the challenge of puberty, are a time when an imbalance can have particularly catastrophic consequences.

Daniel is just one of many young people who, through no fault of his own, began to go off course because a serious imbalance developed in his brain. When, as an eight-month-old fetus, Daniel was in danger of being forced down the birth canal too soon, his brain simply reacted instinctively. Was this reaction helpful to Daniel? Certainly—it possibly saved his life. But was it helpful when he grew up? No, it was entirely unhelpful, and in fact became the reason he lost his way and was unaware of his potential to be a robust and happy individual.

Thankfully, through brain training, Daniel had incredible success breaking his dominant overactive parasympathetic pattern—the freeze pattern. When he balanced his brain, the way he looked and even the way he talked and walked changed immediately. His academic performance improved dramatically, and his smile and natural warmth filled the space around him. His ability to connect with himself enabled him to feel more connected with others, which opened the door for people to associate with him. Soon he was hanging out with good friends like any normal kid.

2

What Really Drives
Dysfunctional Behavior?

THERE ARE COUNTLESS CASES ON RECORD of individuals who showed no trace of antisocial behavior and were even model citizens, who suddenly went on a rampage, in some cases killing their own family and in other cases slaughtering people where they worked or attended school.

"He was such a mild-mannered man," people often say of the individual who turns a gun on his wife and children. "How can this have happened?"

Take the case of Steven Kazmierczak. In February 2008, he wrote a note to his girlfriend asking her not to forget him, then burst onto the stage of an Illinois campus lecture hall with guns blazing. If there is such a thing as a profile of a mass murderer, Kazmierczak didn't seem to fit it. He was an outstanding student, courteous, industrious, and had a promising future in criminal justice ahead of him.

After the twenty-seven year old stopped taking his medication for depression, his behavior became erratic. Two weeks later, he gunned down students at his former college. Researchers discovered his friendly exterior masked a troubled mind. It turns out that, in his teens, Kazmierczak used to cut himself.

Again, the sympathetic nervous system is akin to the gas pedal in an automobile, whereas the parasympathetic functions more like the brake pedal. In each second of our existence, the sympathetic and parasympathetic are both at work, applying the gas pedal and the brake in exactly the right order and proportions to keep our body functioning at a level optimized to whatever we are doing at any given moment.

The sympathetic nervous system incites both activity and emotion. But if the parasympathetic becomes dominant, it can suppress the ability to act, as well as the ability to feel.

Being unable to feel can cause self-destructive tendencies to mandate an experience of feeling, even driving a person to cut themselves.

It's most likely Kazmierczak was so parasympathetic-dominant that he experienced a freeze response, and one way out of this locked-down state was to cut himself in an attempt to feel something.

How a "Nice" Person Turns Rogue

If the parasympathetic acts as a brake and is associated more with "stop" than "go," why would a person whose parasympathetic is strongly dominant plan to harm others?

To answer this, we have to rethink some of society's most commonly held beliefs about how violence is triggered.

When an individual's suppressed aggression isn't addressed, the brain will find other ways, depending on the intensity of the aggression, to attempt to mitigate the imbalance. A teen may join a gang. The brain is also likely to induce them to use alcohol or drugs to release their inhibitions, allowing the suppressed aggression to be anesthetized briefly. It's like giving the uncomfortable brain a shot of Novocain.

This is one reason college students, away from parental control perhaps for the first extended period in their lives, are particularly notorious for the excessive amount of alcohol they consume. It's also likely why so many "good" kids get into trouble in their teens. Thankfully, a vast majority of our young people pass through this phase without serious incident. But when there is a severe imbalance in the brain and it is stuck in one dominant pattern, the course is set for the person to end up in real trouble. With the brake all the way on, they may become dissociated from reality, as was beginning to happen with Daniel in the last chapter and did in fact happen with Steven Kazmierczak.

It's a natural response for the brain to dissociate from an event when it is trying to protect itself. For instance, dissociation often happens to people when they are in auto accidents. They describe everything that's happening to them as "slowed down." This is because the brain recognizes a crash is coming and dissociates itself from the incident in an attempt to survive. It knows that if the neurons are banged together, they will experience shock. Therefore, the axons and the dendrites—the connectors for the neurons—actually start to separate, pulling apart in order to defend themselves. This is why everything appears to take place in slow motion.

In the state of dissociation, a person simply isn't in touch with the real world. In the case of a heavy sympathetic dominance, where the gas pedal is stuck in the on position, the individual is driven by a need to be in constant motion. This person, who is typically overly competitive and easily angered, will often shift to another activity even before the current task is complete.

"They Know Not What They Do"

When dissociation occurs, the individual tends to experience what they are doing as if someone else were doing it. Yet, unaware as they may be of what they are doing, they are driven to do it just the same. They have such a strong need to experience feelings that they will go to extremes to satisfy this need. So what we have is an intensely emotional person committing an impulsive act of which they have no real awareness because they are caught up in the emotion.

Dissociation is one reason people are able to commit incredibly violent acts such as gunning down a fellow student or, in the case of an unwelcomed divorce, killing their former spouse and even their own children. The reality is they truly do not know what they are doing at the time.

A person whose brain is subjected to life-threatening trauma may learn not to feel. They don't *choose* not to feel. Rather, the brain automatically shuts down their capacity to feel or experience emotion. This is the brain's way of getting them through what they have experienced. It's purely a survival tactic.

At the same time, the brain seeks balance, and consequently the person may actually have a longing to feel. If the desire to feel builds up sufficiently, the person may try flooring their gas pedal— or, in other words, revving up their sympathetic nervous system. This desperate attempt to feel something is a misguided attempt to counteract the individual's state of utter emotional numbness. An extremely dangerous situation has now developed.

As the person makes a move intended to induce feeling, paradoxically the brain resists, based on its painful experiences from the past—the same experiences that caused it to shut down its ability to feel in the first place. The brain now senses that to feel will be too painful. So while the individual is trying to floor their gas pedal in order to counteract their brake, the brain pushes even harder on its brake. In other words, the brain is fighting itself.

We now have a situation in which the person is pushing hard to feel, while the brain, sensing its survival is threatened, is working equally hard to keep the feelings down. The result can be that the person acts but never actually experiences the feelings they were seeking.

The brain has separated the person from the act they are engaged in. In fact, the person no longer even sees themselves in that activity. It's as if they take on another identity. In such a situation, things can go completely awry, as in a campus shooting or the killing of one's own family.

Often, when it's all over, the perpetrator can't believe they did what they did. They may now see the results of their actions and be equally as horrified as everyone else. This is how an individual no one could imagine committing such a terrible act ends up shooting other human beings. The perpetrator has truly broken their link to reality during their violence.

The dissociation that arises in such an incident produces a frozen state. It's as if the person has been stored in a freezer, so that their body begins to ice, yet they are still alive on the inside. Beyond a certain point, the person doesn't realize that they are being frozen because their brain cuts off the body's senses so it won't feel the pain anymore. The situation is parallel to when someone falls through the ice on a pond and can't save themselves. The brain tells the body to shut down, completely dissociating itself from the body and its environment in order to keep itself alive as long as possible in the hope of rescue.

Consider the case of a pet tropical fish left in the care of family while its owner was away on vacation. When the day came to return the fish, the weather was extremely hot, so the aquarium was placed in an ice chest in the trunk of the car. When the chest was opened at its destination, the fish was found floating, apparently dead from the cold as it was accustomed to being in warm water. But what if the fish might still be alive? The water was warmed ever so slowly so as not to shock the fish, just in case it was still living. Slowly, the fish started to move. The brain's survival strategy had worked. Sadly, humans in a state of frozen dissociation commit acts that too often don't promote life but instead result in tragedy for themselves and perhaps others.

In our courts of law, we hold people responsible for their actions. Unless they are shown to be insane, we regard them as responsible people who should have known better. But when a person floors their gas pedal to counteract a brake stuck in the on position, and then finds themselves in a frozen state, such an action isn't coming from responsible logic, it's coming from an imbalance in the brain.

In such an instance, we can understand more fully why Jesus said of his executioners: "They know not what they do."

3

Searching for Ourselves in
All the Wrong Places

IN MODERN SOCIETY, humans tend to become focused on activities.
We talk a great deal about what we are *doing* and our achievements.
Simply *being* isn't our forte. If we were to describe most people, we
should perhaps more accurately speak of them as human *doings*
instead of human *beings*.

When we do enter into the state of just being, our focus shifts
away from activity. Instead, it naturally gravitates to *observing*. This
is because we are born watchers.

As watchers, the person we are most meant to watch is *ourselves*.

When we're no longer in touch with the stillness within our own
being, instead of watching ourselves, we often pay to watch a select
group of "stars" that can do extraordinary things. We adulate actors
and actresses, sports figures, models, and other entertainers, paying
them a fortune. How are they able to command such high figures?

The reason stars make so much money is that we not only like watching, but we can't *help* watching these highly paid icons. Our stargazing culture is a reflection of how desperate we are, because we are so busy doing, to simply *observe*—and of how very much we want to be distracted so that we avoid observing *ourselves*, lest we realize how far short we are falling from our limitless potential.

The Role of Role Models

Is there a place for public role models? There is indeed, as long as the role model acts as a mirror to help us awaken to our own potential. But the mirror can't be distorted if it's going to serve this purpose.

In the early days of television, the mirrors offered to children were the Lone Ranger, Rin Tin Tin, Lassie, the Cisco Kid, Bonanza, Wyatt Earp, and later, Superman. The focus of such heroes was on doing the fair thing, rescuing the downtrodden, helping the oppressed, and saving people who were being victimized. Children saw their own potential in these heroes and wanted to be just like them.

Today, the focus has shifted. We are no longer interested in the character portrayed, but in the portrayer of the character. Our attention is no longer on "the good" versus "the bad," but on the personal lives of performers, many of whose behavior is dysfunctional. Sadly, a whole industry has developed around our enthrallment with these people, supplying us with endless tabloid gossip, invasive photos from paparazzi who hover around stars' every move—and all of this for lucrative sums because our insatiable need for images commands it.

As we watch the lives of the rich, the royal, and the famous on television, in the movies, at the sports arena, or in the tabloids, we tell ourselves they are more special than ourselves. By treating stars like an aristocracy, society reinforces this message. At the same time, we buy the tabloids to reassure ourselves the celebrity is actually no better than we are. In fact, there is a direct relationship between how well a person is doing in terms of their own happiness and contentment, and how likely they are to buy a tabloid. Gawking at the tabloids is a way of affirming that our brain's "screwedupness" is okay. What a cycle! All of this is keeping us from seeing our own limitless possibilities.

When a person becomes famous, they hold a special place in society, which carries with it a responsibility. If the famous, in their egotism, forsake their potential to be effective mirrors for us, they forsake *us*. They mess up our potential. The famous person who, aware that millions are watching them, says, "I can do whatever I want," then behaves in a manner that's less than wholesome, lets us down. At the very moment they have an opportunity to show us our potential, they fail us. If we lack an awareness of our worth, we find ourselves identifying with society's superstars regardless of their atrocious behavior. This is a vicious cycle, because all the while we are watching others, it's really *our own authentic self* we are searching for—a self found in our inner *being*.

Awakening to Ourselves Through Our Reflection in Others

How greatly we are affected by other people, who can either limit our ability to see our own essential being or serve as a mirror to show us our potential, can be seen in the case of Karen, who, when she was a young girl, was told repeatedly that she was stupid and would never amount to anything.

Now a thirty-four-year-old single woman, Karen is insecure, shy, and in many ways withdrawn. Because she learned to think of herself in a minimal way, she restricts her participation in life to activities that feel "safe" to her and that fall within her vision of her own potential.

Karen's shyness stems from a pattern that became more and more deeply etched into her brain each time she was told she would never make anything of herself. Her brain perceived this view of herself as a threat. In order to minimize this threat, her brain adopted a protective mode, which caused Karen to behave in ways that avoided drawing attention to herself.

Karen's brain perceived that if she tried to excel at anything, she would only be criticized. Out of sheer self-preservation, her brain caused her to make herself as invisible as possible. So Karen lives her life with the idea that if no one notices her, no one will find fault with her.

In other words, the parasympathetic dominance Karen's brain used in childhood to protect her from a potential barrage of criticism has become her Achilles' heel now that she's a grown woman. But this protective pattern no longer serves her well because she has no real friends, and the idea of being in a romantic relationship is simply beyond the scope of her imagination. She tells herself, "Who would want someone like me?"

One morning as Karen orders her daily cup of latte at Starbucks, the person taking her order remarks, "Some of our customers are in such a rush. They are demanding and complain a lot, but you are always so pleasant!"

Karen has never thought of herself as pleasant. On the contrary, she thinks of herself as socially inept. But just the fact that she caught someone's eye—that someone noticed her—has a profound emotional impact on her self-worth. It opens a window to an entirely different view of herself.

How did the Starbucks server's simple statement, "You are

always so pleasant!" have such a profound impact on Karen when their contact with each other was so fleeting?

When a person's sense of themselves has suffered at the hands of one individual, it's equally the case that a different individual can impact this person's brain pattern in a positive way. Once this happens, negative neural connections that have existed for years can begin to rewire.

It isn't so much the factual information in the Starbucks server's statement that presents Karen with the chance to see herself differently. It's the emotional impact of the statement that draws her out. The encounter awakens the chemical factory within her brain, and this chemical factory holds the possibility of changing the patterns of shyness already etched into her neural network.

In each of our encounters with our fellow humans, we all have an opportunity to affect another person's life either positively or negatively. We either reinforce brain patterns that no longer serve, or we act as a mirror of the person's potential that opens the way for an entirely new vision of themselves to emerge.

The kind of interaction that took place between Karen and the Starbucks attendant also takes place when a person goes to a psychotherapist or other professional counselor, only in a more focused form. The synergy is identical. It's not so much what the therapist knows that makes a difference in a client's life, nor the particular modality the therapist uses. It's really the relationship between the therapist and the client that drives the whole therapeutic experience. A skillful counselor mirrors the client in such a manner that the individual can see themselves more clearly. To the degree that a counselor is unable to do this, the counseling works less successfully.

Studies have shown that therapy works about as well as a really good friend. This is because, in all our experiences, we seek to see ourselves. That we seek to see ourselves in our many experiences and encounters with others may not be obvious at first. For instance, if we develop a good friendship, it's because we seek companionship, someone to talk to who understands us, and someone who values us. But why do we resonate with this person?

Suppose you are five years old and go to the playground. Of all the children playing there, which one do you gravitate toward? Someone like yourself. When we tell someone, "I like you," what are we really saying? We are saying that in some significant way they are like us and we are like them.

A good friend is somebody who in certain key ways is like ourselves. We are drawn to a particular individual because we see in them qualities we celebrate in ourselves. We are also drawn to people because they have qualities we wish we had.

In other words, the person functions as a mirror for us. We see ourselves in this individual.

Being able to observe ourselves is what allows our essential *being* to express itself, enabling us to move toward our potential. We may not be consciously aware of this, but intuitively we each know that if we can but see ourselves, we will recognize our potential, gain clarity, and know where to go with our life and how to get there.

Getting Ourselves in Focus

The brain is focused on keeping itself alive because this is its primary task. In fact, it has served us so well in this capacity over the years that it's satisfied with just keeping us alive. This is why so many of us endure the monotony of mediocre lives, content with the mundane.

However, the brain isn't who we are: it's a tool we use. For this reason, life continually invites us to pull our head out of the sand

and look around for a mirror in which to discover our possibilities beyond mere survival. It seeks to open us up to our limitless being.

When the server at Starbucks told Karen, "You are so pleasant," it caused Karen to pull her head out of the sand. In fact, it gave her such a lift that she looks forward to seeing this same server every morning when she orders her coffee. In spite of all she heard about herself growing up and has repeated to herself all these years, her deepest being resonates with what the server says. She longs to hear that she is a wonderful person, and so going to Starbucks becomes something to which she looks forward. She enjoys the rapport she has with the person who makes her latte because she is glimpsing her real self. This is because, no matter how negatively we may have seen ourselves for most of our life and no matter how limited the view of ourselves wired into our brain, at some deep intuitive level each of us knows we possess intrinsic value and limitless potential.

What happens when, one morning, someone else is behind the counter at Starbucks, someone with whom Karen experiences no synergy? When she enters the building and notices the usual attendant isn't present, Karen's heart sinks. Why? Nothing about Karen has changed. She is the same person buying the same latte she has purchased every morning in the past. Her heart sinks because she is experiencing how much she wants to be noticed. She longs to see herself in the mirror of another person who likes her—someone who is in some measure *like* her.

When Karen finds herself confronted with a different server, she feels a little lost and doesn't quite know what to do with herself. To cope with the awkwardness she is experiencing, she fumbles around in her purse while the attendant fixes her latte. In a very real sense, Karen has lost sight of herself because the mirror that showed her to herself is no longer available.

When we don't have a mirror to reflect back to us our "okay-ness," we become anxious. We become focused on *doing* instead of *being*. The reason for this is that doing helps us escape the fact we don't feel good about ourselves. By keeping ourselves busy, we don't have to ponder our life. But the price is that we lose our center of gravity.

Quantum physics teaches us that observation plays a role in what becomes actualized in our world because there is an inter-play between the observer and the observed. For this reason, we are dependent on everyone, and everyone is dependent on us. Because we are interdependent in terms of how we develop as indi-viduals, we yearn for someone to mirror back to us what a mag-nificent person we really are. It's wonderful when mirroring happens. Someone says, "You are so nice," and all at once we have a fresh image of ourselves. We are seeing ourselves in a way we haven't seen ourselves until now. Such mirroring awakens a love of ourselves and, in turn, a love of each other. We are seeing what we *can* be—what our potential is.

Mirror, Mirror on the Wall

Wonderful as it is to find in another person a mirror that awakens us to ourselves, this can only serve to kick-start our journey toward the flourishing of our limitless potential. It cannot take us very far because, as long as we look to others for a sense of identity, we experience only a borrowed sense of self.

For example, we buy the same shoes, the same lipstick, and the same designer outfits because we need so desperately to feel like we are "someone." Though such an identity transfusion may keep us going for a time, ultimately it fails us. Faced with this failure, which may take the form of a midlife crisis, a divorce, losing our job, a deep unhappiness with the status quo of our life, or such a simple thing as a server not showing up at Starbucks, we are invited to recognize and embrace our *own* uniqueness.

In an era when many role models seem increasingly to focus on their own narcissistic pursuits as if they were a cut above everybody else and no longer carry out the task of mirroring our potential, it's especially imperative we switch our focus from the *external* world to our *own inner being*.

But how are we to do this? How can we become an effective observer of our own self?

4

The Brain Becomes Its Own Mirror

THE ART OF TRAINING ONE'S BRAIN is ancient. To train the brain by enabling it to become its own mirror is akin to what people have practiced for thousands of years through meditation.

Why are we drawn to meditation? Because it leads us to the deep state of being that lies beneath our mental chatter and emotional reactivity.

During meditation, we are in the role of a watcher. We become an observer of our thoughts, emotions, moods, and intents. Perhaps we use a mantra or focus on our breathing as a way to quiet our mind. Alternatively, we may place our attention on how our body feels or bring awareness to a particular part of our body such as our hands, chest, or stomach. There are a variety of forms of meditation, but each in their different way can bring us to the contented state that's bedrock to our being.

The point of meditation is to enable the brain to quiet itself. As the brain becomes calmer, in some way it is then able to rebalance itself. Instead of clinging to the disturbed patterns it established long ago, it begins adjusting itself to reflect its optimal state.

While meditation can slowly bring this state about, people in western cultures have found it difficult to meditate with the ease that many in eastern cultures do. This is because, from the time we are born until the time we die, westerners adhere to ingrained patterns of human *doing* instead of human *being*. We are so wrapped up in seeking our value through doing that we fail to recognize the true value of simply being. Our entire sense of value may be hitched to what we accomplish by doing.

To focus on *being* doesn't mean we sit on a rock concentrating on our navel. Rather, it means we do what we need to do and want to do, but without deriving our worth from such activities. We experience a fundamental "okayness" about ourselves that isn't determined or validated by accomplishments. A balanced brain has this feel of "okayness," which forms a solid foundation from which to do the things we do. When we have a sense that we are fundamentally okay, we catch onto all kinds of new information about ourselves that was there all the time, though we couldn't recognize it because our unbalanced brain was blocking our vision. For instance, a person who has always felt unattractive suddenly discovers, "Why, I am kinda cute." Or perhaps they realize, "I am quite charming" or "I have a good sense of humor." None of this is new information—it's always been inside us. We are seeing what we have long intuited about ourselves, though we haven't known how to verify it. We are reclaiming our essential self.

Watching and Listening to Ourselves

Because of advancements in technology, today we are able to help the brain see itself in an optimized state much easier and faster than we are generally able to accomplish through meditation. Brain technology has given us the ability to provide a mirror for the brain in a form to which it readily responds.

Let me share with you how this technology came about, because then you will better understand how it works. I was struggling with post-traumatic stress disorder during a difficult period in my life. I had gone to many different health practitioners in my attempt to free myself from the symptoms of this disorder, but nothing proved effective.

My career at the time required that my brain go back and forth between two fundamentally different functions, which meant continually switching between using the detailed and analytical area of my brain and using the creative and contextual area of my brain. It was while I was struggling with this challenge that I was introduced to biofeedback. My frustration with needing to repeatedly switch from one side to the other, coupled with continued symptoms of post-traumatic stress, pushed me to go deeply into biofeedback and later neurofeedback. I went to various schools to learn how these modalities worked, as well as consulting with several gurus in different parts of the world.

There are some exceptionally bright, capable people in biofeedback and neurofeedback, and it was the talent of several of them that paved the way for brain training to emerge. In terms of how the brain works, I especially garnered a great deal of insight from the neurofeedback specialists.

In biofeedback, and particularly neurofeedback, I at last began to find clues to how I might end my misery. But although biofeedback and neurofeedback both helped me to see that I could heal, I soon realized this was going to require far too much time. Working exceptionally long hours in an anxious state, I was already easily angered and somewhat distracted, which meant I wasn't much fun to be around, to which my two grown children can attest. To add countless hours of neurofeedback to my schedule was more than I could manage. Perhaps I would have done it in hundreds of sessions were I suffering from an injury that caused me to lack functionality, but as a fairly functional person, I needed to solve my problems without creating a new one by cramping my time even more.

It's said that necessity is the mother of invention. I certainly had a specific personal need, and this led me to become inventive. Being neither a medical doctor nor a neuroscientist, but a computer software designer with a background in both psychology and theology, I was fascinated by how computers might help people get their lives back.

I wanted my own life back! Following years of analysis after succumbing to post-traumatic stress, I realized none of this was allowing me to go on with my life. Was it just me? Was I too hardheaded to let go of my trauma? Or had I simply not found a method that could release me from the emotional chaos and hypervigilance in which I was trapped?

Neurofeedback attempts to change a behavior by showing us how our neural network is functioning. We then endeavor to change our behavior. I pondered my own post-traumatic stress in light of this, and the question that came to me was: If we can voluntarily change our brain functioning over an extended period of time by noticing what needs to change and applying a technique such as neurofeedback to help us make the change, could there be a shorter way of achieving this from which practically anyone could benefit?

I took into account everything I had learned about neurofeedback, coupled with my understanding of the capabilities of computers and my insights from psychology and theology, then applied an overarching approach to this information. The approach was born out of the basic insight of quantum physics, which, as mentioned earlier, postulates that when something is observed, it is changed by the act of being observed. This is the key to how brain training works.

Brain training shows the brain a mirror of itself in an optimized state. How does showing the brain itself in an optimized state work? It's not unlike the way we use a mirror to improve our appearance. Each morning, countless men peer into a mirror to shave. The mirror allows them to spruce up their appearance without cutting themselves. Similarly, women use a mirror to do their hair in the morning, then carry a mirror in their purse all day because it's difficult to put on lipstick without one. Looking at ourselves allows us to make changes to our appearance.

Observing ourselves is helpful in a variety of other ways. For instance, if a golfer watches a video of their swing, they can sometimes see a problem they are having and change it. Athletes of all kinds use video these days to enable themselves to gain an edge in their sport. This is also why we have coaches and even sometimes psychotherapists. They act as a kind of mirror, showing us how to improve our stride in a race, how to handle a ball more effectively, or how to make sense of the chaos in our lives.

While a video or a coach may be helpful in sports, they're not much help to someone who is shaving or putting on their makeup. Seeing themselves in real time is infinitely more useful. This is also the case when it comes to altering behavior. For instance, someone who explodes with rage and says things they later regret may be shocked and embarrassed when they watch a video of themselves exhibiting this kind of behavior, and they may then and there determine to make a change, but in practice this usually proves difficult. By the time the next provocation arises, the shock of how they behaved has worn off. Before they know it, they are caught up in a fresh bout of rage. However, were they able to observe themselves in real time—seeing themselves right as they are about to erupt, and simultaneously seeing their brain in an optimized state—they would have a chance to stop their anger in its tracks. As they do this, the brain may create a new pathway, providing a far better alternative to rage.

Our need is for the brain to see itself in a balanced state. A balanced brain leads people to grab onto the potential they already *know* they have—and yet, as we've seen, *don't* know.

Brain training functions as a mirror that enables us to balance our brain. Describing the effect of brain training, one person remarked, "The feeling is one of 'Here I am!' Later, there was the wondering of where have I been all this time?"

By enabling the brain to see itself and balance itself, brain training gives us options from which to choose, rather than a single dominant unhealthy pathway to follow. Perhaps for the first time, we can see who we really are and what we want from life and wish to contribute to the world.

The Brain Learns to Observe Itself

During brain training, the brain's own balanced and harmonized wave patterns are fed back to it so that it can observe itself in a balanced state. How is the brain shown its own energy patterns?

The brain runs on tiny voltages of electricity. A brainwave is electromagnetic energy that can be broken down into frequencies. We measure energy by measuring the peaks and valleys in its modulation (its movement), which we refer to as its frequency. The number of peaks and valleys that occur each second are measured in a unit of measurement called hertz. In other words, one peak and one valley in one second of time is defined as one cycle per second and is a frequency of one hertz. Higher frequencies have more cycles per second and are represented in sound as higher notes on a musical scale, while lower frequencies have fewer cycles per second and are like the lower notes on a musical scale.

To feed the brain's own optimal wave patterns back to it non-invasively, we have to access it through the ears in the form of sound transmitted through stereo headphones. However, if you simply recorded your brain then played it back to yourself in the form of sound, it would be ineffective. The problem is that humans are unable to hear these frequencies via the ears because they are outside our audio range.

During the development of brain training, the challenge was to transfer the frequencies so they are audible and recognizable by the brain as sound waves the brain itself is generating—only then can it interpret them. Fortunately, electrical energy and sound energy are different forms of the same thing—modulation. In fact, the impulses of the central nervous system actually behave more like a sound wave than an electrical wave.

The key turned out to be a set of algorithms that translate brain functions to sound in real time. Before the brain's frequencies can be useful to itself, calculations must be carried out that translate the frequencies to a fraction of a hertz. The result is that when the electrodes detect frequency changes in a person's brain, the frequency changes identically in their ears also.

Why sound instead of a graphics representation on a video monitor? Because with sound, the response time from the brain back to the client takes less than fifty milliseconds, versus 1,250 milliseconds or greater for a graphic representation of a brain function.

When the brain hears the sounds that are transmitted to it, it says to itself, "I'm doing that!" As soon as it picks up on this, changes in the neural network begin to occur. Connections that were formed at one time to protect us, but that no longer serve us well, seem either to disconnect themselves or become non-dominant. Earlier life connections that are more original, healthier connections then begin to create a dominant pattern. As a result, the energy of the brain flows along more beneficial pathways than when it flowed along pathways that were useful at one particular time but now limit us.

Let me restate all of this more simply. When a person's brain is being trained, all that the training is really doing is holding up a mirror in the form of sound to reflect how an unbalanced brain looks at a particular moment in contrast to how a balanced brain might look. During the process of mirroring, an amazing thing happens. The brain not only recognizes that it is hearing its own patterns in the sound it is receiving, it gravitates toward the more balanced pattern that is being provided! Then it adjusts itself until it achieves a flexibility and balance overall. The brain is miraculous after all.

When we show the brain itself, it knows where to adjust itself because it recognizes where the electrodes are placed. Not only is there a small device on the skin in a specific place to advise it, the brain energy that is translated into sound originates from that specific place. Other parts of the brain then balance themselves according to the new balance achieved in the areas specified under the electrodes.

In other words, brain training allows the brain to see itself in an optimized state. It sees only the optimized patterns and gravitates toward those patterns, establishing them as its own dominant patterns. It then recognizes that this is in fact its *natural* state.

Because of this, it is attracted toward this optimized condition like iron filings to a magnet.

How does this happen? I don't know fully, but our evolving understanding of brain plasticity—how the brain isn't a fixed entity, as we used to think, but is able to reorganize itself—is part of the answer. After over 10,000 views of brain energy before and after training, I do know that it works.

Can Brain Training Harm You?

If the brain can spontaneously adjust itself to conform to a clear vision of its authentic state, could brain training ever have a negative impact?

This was a crucial question in my own mind when I first developed the technology. I wanted my son to try it, but first I had to be sure it wouldn't harm him. For instance, I wanted to know whether a person would be more uncomfortable if a less-than-optimized state were shown to the brain instead of an optimized state. To find out, I tested this on myself to see the effects. I secluded myself in a cabin and for a month attempted to train my brain in every way that was the opposite of how I trained it to feel better.

The first time I tried to train myself in a negative fashion, I felt a little uncomfortable for about a half-hour afterwards. Then the discomfort left and I felt like my normal self again. When I again attempted this, the discomfort lasted only a few minutes. On several successive occasions, I experienced nothing at all. Why? It was as if my brain were saying, "I don't like this, and I'm not buying it because it doesn't feel natural."

When the brain isn't stuck in either a sympathetic or parasympathetic dominance, it gravitates toward homeostasis. Training the brain simply helps it remove blockages that keep it from seeking to function in its most natural, optimal manner. Thousands of people have trained their brain on several continents without a single incident of harm done, though temporary discomfort may be possible due to the individual experiencing new feelings that are unfamiliar to them. On the contrary, positive reports continually flood in from people who have had truly life-changing results.

If training can't be used to corrupt the brain, can it be used to generate skills an individual doesn't naturally possess? For instance, could a person without natural musical ability train their brain and become a concert pianist?

Since musical ability isn't alien to the brain's natural state, it's possible this could be done. But the person would have to do a great deal of brain training and also practice at the keyboard tens of thousands of hours. The reason for this is that we each have unique neural networks. If a person doesn't have the required natural ability, they clearly don't have a neural network that lends itself to musical expression. Even a person with the right network has to practice and practice, and about three-quarters of those who aspire to be concert pianists quit after 2,000 to 3,000 hours of practice.

When a person with no natural talent practices the piano, they are trying to inscribe a pattern into their neural network. They are working *from the outside in*. Brain training works best in the opposite direction, helping the faculties already present in the brain's networks to function more effectively so that the person's inherent aptitude can find expression. In other words, it works *from the inside out*. It's successful because it goes with one's natural predisposition and adds flexibility.

5

In Search of a Contented Brain

IN WHAT WAYS IS BRAIN TRAINING similar and dissimilar to biofeed-back and neurofeedback? It's a question people often ask.

Biofeedback and neurofeedback are both helpful modalities, and, as we have seen, both played a role in the development of brain training. However, there are significant differences not only in the technique used in the kind of brain training known as Brain State Conditioning™, but also in the array of imbalances it can address.

Biofeedback dates back to the 1960s. It works by raising a person's awareness of what's happening in their body. The information is gleaned from monitoring devices placed on the skin at various points on the body to garner data about muscle tension, heart rate, skin temperature, and sweat gland activity. The information is then shared with the individual so that they get a snapshot of how they respond to various situations that are presented to them.

In other words, biofeedback works much like using a thermometer to detect a fever, then responding to the information with appropriate steps to help the body fight the fever. Or we might liken it to using a bathroom scale to detect weight gain or loss, then responding to the information through diet, exercise, and so on.

Although the autonomic nervous system is usually thought of as something we don't have much control over, a person who is made aware of their bodily state can in fact alter certain aspects of the nervous system, such as heart rate and blood pressure. This can be helpful because it allows a person to gain a measure of control over the functioning of their autonomic nervous system. To accomplish this, the individual learns to observe what's happening in their body and how to respond to it in a constructive way.

For instance, a person who experiences panic attacks can use biofeedback to observe how their heart rate quickens as the panic comes on. In their biofeedback training sessions, they are able to see exactly what happens to their temperature, blood pressure, sweat glands, and other bodily systems while they focus on a particular issue with which they are dealing. The ability to focus and pay attention to what happens in their body must then transfer to their everyday life, in which no biofeedback instruments are available to inform them of what's happening in their chemistry. This requires that the individual become an astute observer of themselves, noticing for instance when they are beginning to sweat or their muscles are becoming tense. By paying attention to how their biology is changing, they are alerted when an unhelpful reaction has begun. With coaching, people can teach themselves to gradually lessen the intensity of their reactions.

An Advancing Technology

In the early days of biofeedback, scientists hoped for spectacular results through increased knowledge of the body. Perhaps, they proposed, we could affect our health in major ways, such as lowering our blood pressure by increasing our awareness of our body chemistry, which would mean drugs would no longer be required. Maybe we could greatly increase our talent, too, by simply becoming more aware of ourselves and the ways in which we tend to excel. Although biofeedback hasn't totally lived up to the more expansive dreams to which it was once linked, it continues to be helpful in cases of stroke-induced paralysis, for relieving migraine and tension headaches, and for helping people cope with anxiety, insomnia, digestive disorders, cardiac arrhythmia, Raynaud's disease, epilepsy, chronic pain, and urinary incontinence. In fact, one study showed it can reduce incontinence by up to 94%. Biofeedback has also proven helpful in pain management.

Neurofeedback grew out of biofeedback, which in turn grew out of our ability to monitor EEG patterns. The technique originated in experiments carried out by NASA to explore the effects of weightlessness on astronauts in outer space.

Neurofeedback recognizes the brain as the control center of the body, which drives our various biological systems. Data is collected from the client's brain and a video monitor is used to display brainwaves. The individual draws on the data gleaned from the brain to see where the brain's functioning is less than optimal. Then the information is used to make changes to how the brain performs. By learning to pay attention, it's possible to increase certain frequencies of brainwaves and decrease other frequencies. This requires considerable effort on the part of the client, who has to be very focused—a task that's especially difficult for someone with an attention deficit disorder. Sound or visual effects are then used to reward the brain when it responds in a beneficial manner. Sometimes games are used to help the person focus and provide a means of feedback.

There are thousands of neurofeedback providers around the world and they have seen their endeavors supported by success across a wide range of pathologies. However, the protocols have never been standardized and consequently there hasn't been a way for providers to collect data in a uniform manner so we can see what is really going on when they apply the various methodologies. It's difficult to do any kind of clinical testing of which neurofeedback protocols work and which don't. This is because double-blind testing, which is the standard for clinical testing, doesn't work where brain function is involved. The brain is no dummy, and any attempt to trick it into thinking a placebo is the real thing is both technically difficult and expensive. In other words, neurofeedback is rather like herding cats. The cat is a creature with a mind of its own and doesn't take well to being organized by humans. Because neurofeedback is highly subjective, the only way to know whether a protocol works is to try it on a particular individual.

Neural networks, once deeply etched into the brain, don't readily change. So although neurofeedback is helpful for some people, it's not an easy solution for others. Bringing about change through neurofeedback in a person whose neural pathways are deeply entrenched is in some ways akin to a scene in the movie *Chocolat*, where one of the citizens of a small French town is attempting to learn a catechism. The children in the class have no difficulty learning, but though the older man goes over and over the catechism, he still can't get it right. His neural pathways are so set in concrete that it's difficult for him to introduce new ones.

Practitioners of neurofeedback don't talk about a cure for conditions, but rather seek to help people function better despite their condition.

The Uniqueness of Each Human Brain

The most complex system in the world that we know of is the three-pound mass between our ears. How are we to understand this complex instrument sufficiently to be able to bring about an optimized pattern for it?

For neurofeedback to get the brain to function in its normal state requires some kind of basis for what constitutes a normal brain. To create such an image, neurofeedback practitioners established a database of brain patterns from several thousand people and averaged the patterns to produce a norm. A neurofeedback client's brain pattern is then compared to this norm. In this way, it's possible to identify brain frequencies that are different from those of an average brain.

Though this is a helpful technique, in some ways it's akin to having a plastic surgeon take a picture of your face and then regenerate that photo showing you how your face would look after plastic surgery based on a comparison of your face to an average face. Because we are such unique individuals, the features that look best on one person may not be remotely suited to another. This is why plastic surgeons don't show you a photograph of what your face would look like if it were to be "averaged." They show you what your face would look like if it were specifically sculpted to suit your unique features. For instance, if you have a crooked nose, you can see exactly how your nose will look after it has been straightened.

We are each unique, as borne out by the fact that tens of millions of fingerprints have been studied yet no two have been found to be the same. Think about how much more complicated the brain's patterns are than a fingerprint and you get some idea of how huge the improbability is that one brain is the same as another. Because an individual's brain patterns are as unique as their fingerprints, brain training doesn't try to alter the brain to that of an "average" but seeks to show each individual brain how it might look after regaining its own balance based on mathematical algorithms.

There are a variety of sound therapies, such as biurnal beats, which also attempt to get the brain to move to a particular frequency by feeding different frequencies into each ear. The trouble is, this is like saying that my size shoe will fit you. For this reason, I wouldn't advocate binaural beats for anybody unless I knew exactly in real time that their brain needed a certain frequency. This doesn't mean biurnal beats don't help some people, but most are not going to get the help they need. Some may even become uncomfortable because the brain pattern the biurnal beats are trying to produce is precisely what these individuals already have in excess. In this, biurnal beats are quite different from brain training, which doesn't worsen an imbalance even if we try to get it to do so. This is because biurnal beats are invasive, whereas brain training is only mirroring. Incorrect mirroring isn't accepted by the brain, whereas invasive procedures still have to be received, even to the brain's detriment.

Not only do brains have unique patterns, pathologies don't exhibit the same brainwave footprint. For instance, a person may say they are depressed. In examining the brain assessments of depressed people, sometimes there is a distinct pattern that indicates too much stress, sometimes a pattern that indicates an abundance of fear, sometimes one that indicates a betrayal or loss of connection to the self or others. Yet each of these individuals is "depressed." The reality is that each brain has some similarities to other brains with a similar pathology, but this doesn't limit the pathology to one particular brainwave pattern. There can be dozens of different patterns for any given pathology. How then can one form of medication or one modality be expected to counter all of these patterns?

For the above reasons, brain training doesn't attempt to address a particular pathology. Rather, it recognizes that one size doesn't fit all, and instead of imposing a generalized pattern on the brain, the technology is designed to balance and harmonize each brain individually, which often triggers improvement in a variety of pathologies.

A Contented Brain

Although brain training treats each brain as unique, there had to be a baseline that could serve as a place to begin creating the balancing algorithms that would allow the brain to see itself.

Using a baseline is quite different from averaging the appearance of a brain. To return to the illustration of facial plastic surgery, you need to have some idea of what a face looks like before you start to sculpt a new one. You need to know that it has eyes, a nose, a mouth, a chin, and so on—in other words, that a face looks different from a kneecap or elbow. Similarly, for the brain to see itself in an idealized state requires some sort of idea of what this might look like.

There are people whose lives appear to be balanced. When the various aspects of their lives are balanced, it reflects the fact that the underlying network driving these various aspects is balanced. It's equally the case that when we see people whose behavior is unhealthy, it reflects an imbalance in the neural network. Where does one find a brain sufficiently balanced to serve as a baseline to create algorithms that represent a brain in an ideal state?

One could go to great scientists, great leaders, or great artists. But although such individuals undoubtedly have intriguing brains that enable them to excel in certain aspects of life, it doesn't necessarily mean they have balanced brains.

What's needed is a brain in a state of homeostasis, which is a state in which a person exudes *contentment*. For this purpose, two Buddhist monks, both masters from Tibet, were chosen to determine the baseline of what a balanced brain looks like.

Again, let me emphasize that to select a brain pattern that's a picture of contentment is different from selecting patterns based on thousands of brains and then averaging those patterns. The average brain isn't close to being as balanced as a brain in a state of deep contentment, and consequently averaging even a large number of such brains won't show us what a contented brain looks like.

Helping the Brain Balance Itself

In neurofeedback, the individual is fed information about what's happening in their brain, and they then attempt to bring their brain in line with an average brain. In contrast, brain training doesn't depend on the client to make any attempt to change their brainwave patterns. Instead of relying on the individual's personal effort, brain training invites them to relax and allow their brain to function in a variety of different states.

A brain assessment evaluates the brain in various states, each of which yield different data. In a state of deep relaxation, the brain receives greatly reduced input. Additionally, there is a state in which the client is asked to perform specific tasks to activate the brain lobes being measured. The task state can generate a great deal of input, especially if the person is working on a complex task such as reading or math.

In the actual brain training that follows an assessment, some protocols require the eyes to be open, whereas others work with the eyes closed. In each of these states, the aim is to get the brain to see itself the way it would look were it functioning optimally, regardless of the state in which it is currently operating. To facilitate this, the individual is encouraged to let go of attempting to change their brain. Instead, the brain is helped by the technology to see itself in an ideal state, which empowers it to change itself.

There is a considerable difference between showing the brain itself in an optimized state and helping a client modify behavior through learning new ways to think, feel, and act. Brain training can be efficacious even if a client falls asleep, as it has little to do with learned behavior. It has to do with the brain's ability to see itself, which to some degree can be achieved without the client's participation. Of course, it's always more efficient to have the client participate, but it isn't mandatory. For example, clients adversarial to training, such as those with adolescent misbehavior or antisocial behavior, can be assisted to achieve greater homeostasis even though they are antagonistic to the process but have been manipulated by a parent or mandated by the justice system to try it (even if their intention is nothing other than to have some time out of their cell!).

The value of a brain training system that doesn't require talk therapy or a particular focus on the condition a client seeks to change is made clear in a letter from a military man:

> I served two tours as a Squad Leader and combat infantry-man in Afghanistan, and was diagnosed with post-traumatic stress disorder upon returning home. After two years of intensive group and individual counseling, I was still experiencing many symptoms of the disorder; mainly lack of sleep, irritability, and a high level of anxiety. After Brain State Conditioning, I'm now sleeping better than I ever have, and I am happy to say that my irritability and anger are gone. The

anxiety I previously experienced is now in my control, meaning that I understand my own frustration and can take effective measures to resolve issues, minimizing stress and anxiety. The best part of this technology is that I never had to mention a thing about my combat experiences as this is not a 'talk therapy' solution. I am currently taking a full course load at school and maintaining my family life with a great deal of enjoyment and ease.

Let me also share with you a case that demonstrates how brain training can often help a person even when they can do nothing to help themselves, as told by her father, a doctor of dental science:

Recently my daughter was given a poor-to-hopeless prognosis by a psychiatrist to ever have a normal, productive, happy life. She was diagnosed with paranoid schizophrenia. She heard voices and had visual hallucinations. After brain training, she has not had any audio or visual artifacts, as I call them. She has been completely off any medication and is scheduled for scuba lessons with me, and will begin cosmetology school soon and is planning to finish her B.S. in healthcare sciences, of which she only had thirty-five hours to complete before all the trouble came. Your research and development of brain training has given our family hope for a bright future. Our daughter is twenty-three and now has positive thinking and does not fixate on the past or stay frozen in fear of the future. Thank you for giving us back our daughter.

Empty Headed and Spaced Out

How does the brain accomplish changes without requiring a great deal of effort on our part?

The answer lies in the insights of quantum mechanics. The philosophical difference between a Newtonian approach to matter and a quantum approach cannot be stressed too strongly.

In the Newtonian approach to the cosmos, scientists saw the stuff of the universe—atoms and molecules—as objects that had a distinct existence and that acted upon and reacted to each other. The quantum approach is radically different in that it looks at how everything in the universe is dependent on everything else. In a quantum view of the world, the most profound part of reality isn't the small bit of matter that is seen; rather, it lies in the space that isn't seen. The most important and largest part of existence is the energy and information that lies between particles, rather than the particles themselves. In this view, the particles are almost trivial. It's the relationship between them that's crucial.

Consider a proton, which resides in the nucleus of an atom. This nucleus is orbited by an electron. Were we to make the proton the size of a basketball and the electron the size of a softball, how far apart do you suppose the basketball and the softball would be? Would they be arm's length perhaps? A football field? In fact, the electron's orbit would be twenty miles away.

In the Newtonian view of the world, the proton and electron are the focus of our attention. But in a quantum universe, it's the twenty miles between them that's relevant. The space between the proton and electron contains energy in the form of information. This information drives the universe and makes up virtually all of what we know to be matter.

This isn't an easy concept for us to grasp. People in the East can wrap their head around it more easily than we in the West because they are accustomed to thinking of the emptiness out of which the universe emerges as the really significant aspect of the equation. But it's the information holding the proton and the electron together in the "empty" space that makes brain training possible.

In order to develop protocols for training, the focus isn't on what neurons are doing. Nor is the focus on the dendrites and axons, which are the arms of the neurons, by means of which they connect. These arms make up what's commonly called "white matter," in contrast to the "grey matter" that forms the neurons themselves. Brain training regards a neuron, with its dendrites and axons, as simply a node, which is a means of exchanging information rather like a switch that allows a train to change tracks. In the brain, we try to make these switching points work at an optimal level so that the network functions well. What matters is the vast amount of information being passed, the patterns this information generates, and the flexibility the brain demonstrates while moving from state-to-state.

Brain training measures the information in the spaciousness of the brain, examining the electromagnetic energy the brain uses as it performs various tasks. It's the information within this energy stream that influences how the neurons connect and how patterns are formed. The issue is made more complex by the presence of non-neuronal glial cells, in particular supporting astrocytes and myelin-producing oligodendrocytes. These cells directly impact the transmission of nerve impulses, which is a function of neurons.

Picture strands of seaweed floating in an ocean and being moved by the ocean's currents—the ocean's energy. When the brain's energy shifts, the neurons receive new information that causes them to disconnect from where they are presently anchored and connect in new patterns that improve the functioning of the network.

Given we are mostly space filled with energy, it's the energy flow within this space that we want to change if we are to achieve homeostasis. Working with this space and the energy that flows through it is best accomplished by allowing *the brain itself* to make the changes, rather than attempting to manipulate the neural network to a previously determined state based on what an "average" brain looks like.

6

The Miracle of A New Vision of Yourself

WHEN OUR BRAIN IS IN BALANCE, we find ourselves thinking about possibilities we would never have considered in the past. Indeed, we entertain options for our life we wouldn't have thought realistic before.

Not only does a balanced brain generate thoughts, ideas, imagination, and feelings that are tailored to our unique individuality, our brain is now able to have a major impact on what we can absorb and how effectively we use what we learn. Hence, it empowers us to accomplish goals we previously thought impossible.

People find they blossom when their brain is balanced. Ideas begin coming to them that they would have dismissed in the past. They recognize their potential. They are seeing what they have always known to be true and couldn't get their arms around. It was like a thousand-pound marshmallow they couldn't lift. Now that the information isn't coming from *outside*, but from *inside*, it's as if that thousand-pound marshmallow has been dehydrated and they can put it in their pocket and take it wherever they want to go.

A Case of Severe Impairment

To illustrate how brain training works from the inside out by capitalizing on the brain's most natural state, let me share with you Justin's experience of training his brain.

Justin was born with the umbilical cord wrapped around his neck multiple times. His limbs had limited development and even his voice box was limited. Imagine a brain trying to keep itself alive in a state when it is starved for food and oxygen.

Later, as a young boy, Justin developed a severe case of cerebral palsy. Although he couldn't move his lower body and lacked controlled movement of his upper body, he was able to move himself somewhat when on the floor.

Thankfully, Justin's mother didn't give up on him. She taught him to speak, and although his speech was slow and difficult to understand at times, his language skills allowed him to communicate. However, his vision was severely limited, as both his close-up and distance vision were missing due to the lack of focus caused by his eye movement.

As Justin developed, he became too large physically for his mother to handle. When he was about nineteen, his mother remarried. Her new husband was often called upon to assist her in moving Justin from the floor to the bed and into his wheelchair.

Around this time, Justin became increasingly aware of his limitations and the burden he placed on everyone around him. Shortly after his mother's wedding, he started experiencing so much frustration that it led to outbursts of anger. He began throwing things, becoming verbally abusive, and sometimes lashed out physically at the person who was trying to lift him. These outbursts were followed by great remorse and an emotional meltdown of uncontrollable sobbing.

His mother's relentless dedication to her son, including the belief that somewhere, someone could help Justin, led her to brain training. At the time, Justin was twenty-three. At first he resisted and had to be practically dragged along. But their home life had reached a point where Justin's rage was intolerable. "I used to hit people," he recalls. "I was incredibly cranky because I was so frustrated."

A Change of Perception

The aim of Justin's training was to help his brain observe itself. If it could see itself differently, perhaps his brain could reach a greater state of balance, stimulating new information processing capabilities. For example, one characteristic of Justin's cerebral palsy was that his attention was scattered instead of focused—just like his eyes. Brain training helped him stick with a task and work through the obstacles that arose.

As Justin's ability to participate in life more effectively gathered momentum, his mother commented, "The change in his *perception* of life is changing his life. From the very first brain training session, it was as if *the lens through which he viewed his life* had been replaced with *a different lens*. In fact, it happened to both of us, because I trained right alongside him for a time to help me cope with the situation. As we left the session the first day, we both knew immediately that we were somehow 'different.' After only a few sessions, Justin was no longer lashing out! It still amazes me, because I used to lie in bed at night and say, 'God, please, please help me with Justin. I need a miracle here big time!'"

There was no instant healing of Justin in answer to the cry of his mother's heart. Nevertheless, she got her miracle, though it came in a form she couldn't have anticipated. She explains, "The miracle is in *us*. Justin *is* the miracle. The miracle is *in* him, and it wasn't a one-time shot—it is continuing. The miracle is *the way he has come to see his world in a whole new light.*"

Like everybody else, Justin wanted to be "someone," but until he experienced brain training, he saw himself as pitiful and an obstacle to other people's happiness. After he began training his brain, he saw himself as, in his own words, "simply Justin." It was a profound shift for him, because he simply couldn't do the things other young people do to validate their worth. His worth had to come not from *doing*, but from experiencing his essential *being*.

The miracle occurred as Justin's brain started observing itself. As he began seeing his essence, he was seeing the limitless in himself for the first time. Seeing the creative presence that's both within us and beyond us, Justin became free of the brain chaos that said his physical limitations defined him.

A New Freedom

When Justin's vision of himself changed, his life began lining up in a purposeful direction. He experienced a freedom to pursue the activities he enjoys and the tasks he wants to accomplish without feeling he is up against an impenetrable barrier.

Despite Justin's disability, an energy from beyond his physical resources flows through him and out to the world. Before, it was as if the flow were trying to get through a pipe with a kink in it. Brain training removed the kink. Justin now perceives his life as a flow. His body has responded and is growing more manageable due to this flow. Amazingly, Justin's vision has also improved, and for the first time in his life he can see the mountains that dot the landscape where he lives. Remarkably, he is able to see close-up as well, which means he can read a menu. He is also able to walk with the help of a walker. The *limitless* Justin is slowly taking control of his life.

A classic example of how Justin is now able to transcend his limitations comes from his experience of attending school. Because of the impairment of his eyes, he had never read a book in his life and neither had he written an essay. He got through school and community college because his stepfather and his mother summarized his textbooks for him. When he arrived at community college, because he had a high GPA from high school, he unexpectedly found himself enrolled in an honors class that required him to struggle through books of 500 pages and write essays for examinations. Without the necessary tools to meet this challenge, he scored a D in one of his classes—though he was only a few points from a C. The professor failed to recognize the challenge Justin was facing. But Justin didn't take it personally. Instead, he acquired an electronic version of his textbooks that could read to him, hired a tutor, and became all the more focused on his studies, bringing his grade up to an A.

When many people who don't know Justin see him in a wheelchair, they either avoid him because they don't know how to talk to someone in a wheelchair or they relate to him out of pity. Their narrow focus doesn't allow them to see the unlimited person he really is. But once they get to know him, he becomes the light in their darkness. If you know Justin, you know love and infinite possibility.

Justin's metamorphosis stems from seeing himself as he really is. Realizing that in his essence he is pure love, he sees his world through the eyes of love. He no longer judges himself as inferior or as a victim and no longer fears life's challenges. Instead, he radiates joy and an excitement about life. Whereas he was once angry at the world, today he lights up any room he enters. Indeed, everybody whose life Justin touches is better for having met him.

Justin's story teaches us that the greatest miracle of all is when we "see" that which is around us in a completely different manner—when we embrace a view of our circumstances that's based on limitless love instead of the limitations of fear.

7

A Matter of Balance and Harmony

THE UNIVERSE EXISTS IN A DELICATE BALANCE, ever on a knife-edge. The human brain also exists in a similar fragile balance.

When things are balanced and in harmony, they function better. For example, when the sounds in a musical composition are balanced and in harmony, they make for more enjoyable listening.

Like everything else, for a brain to work well, it should be in a balanced state. In such a state, neither the sympathetic nervous system nor the parasympathetic dominates. The left and right hemispheres of the brain function in tandem. The various lobes on each side of the brain—the brain's neighborhoods—are balanced, and the activities within them are in harmony.

We have already alluded to the fact the lobes of the brain function much like the neighborhoods of a city. In any city there are a variety of neighborhoods. There are industrial neighborhoods where chemicals and raw materials are processed, fuel is refined, trucks and trains arrive and depart around the clock, and there are chemical odors. There are neighborhoods that have a high density of population, which means that a lot of people are crammed into a small space with a number of multi-family dwellings such as condos and apartments. Then there are middle class residential areas as well as palatial estates. All of these neighborhoods have their function, and they are joined by highways that make possible a continuous exchange of goods, services, and relationships.

The neighborhoods of the brain are similar. Each has a unique makeup of varying complexity, each has special tasks to perform, and they are joined by highways that comprise a neural network much like a network of roads or railways in a city. In the same way a person who lives in a residential neighborhood requires gas from the refinery, electricity from the grid, and food from the market, the brain runs on a continual exchange of vital information between its lobes.

In a city, if the functioning of one of the neighborhoods is impaired, it can affect the functioning of the others. For example, a huge fire in an industrial neighborhood can pollute the other neighborhoods, slowing activity to a crawl or even bringing everything to a standstill. A strike by transportation workers in the inner city may mean people from the suburbs can't get to work and shipments of goods don't arrive at their destination on time, affecting the lives of everyone in the city.

Even as the harmonious functioning of each neighborhood in a city is essential to its inhabitants, the human organism functions much more efficiently when its lobes are all in balance, promoting quality of life.

When Life Throws Us a Curve

Many of us suffer from a measure of brain energy imbalance. When this is the case, a difficult period in our lives can exacerbate this imbalance, with unpleasant consequences.

How this happens to perfectly ordinary people who are simply trying to live their lives can be seen in the case of Jane, whose husband developed cancer. For two and a half years, she watched him slowly deteriorate. As she walked down the path toward his death with him, it was not only a heartbreaking experience but also at times frightening. As a consequence, she found herself emotionally and mentally checking out on occasion.

Though Jane felt guilty for needing short periods when she wasn't focused on her husband, the time she took for herself was essential. Although she didn't realize it, she was responding to her brain's need to protect her from an overload.

Whenever we face the death of a loved one, the brain shifts into a protective pattern. It makes no difference whether the death is sudden or whether we find ourselves coping with a lengthy terminal illness. The brain notices we are making too much use of certain neural nets. Overactive neural nets, caused by the high level of energy we are expending on stress and worry, compound our problem because the excess activity stops us from sleeping well. At such times, the brain causes us to dissociate from what's happening in our life. It encapsulates the experience, setting it outside of us as if we weren't actually living it. By so doing, it keeps us from burning out and thereby helps us get through these periods. So although there are times when we need a break from the role of caregiver, this allows us to be helpful to a loved one over a protracted period. If the brain didn't force this on us, we would tend to become so wrapped up in dealing with our own emotional state that we would no longer be able to be present for the other.

Once the trauma is over, the brain pattern established for this purpose is no longer helpful. Still, we find ourselves at times engaged in an activity that reminds us of the time that caused this pattern to arise. It may be something someone says, or looking at a particular scene or photograph and remembering. Before we know it, the painful state comes back to us and floods us. This is because, when we dissociate, the pain is still present even though we aren't focused on it. When it reemerges, it causes tension, often in our joints. If we start to cry, we find ourselves moving into an almost fetal position. A specific brain imbalance is bringing back the pattern of dissociation. When this happens, it's confusing. We might even imagine we are having a breakdown. We think we should be through this problem because it happened so long ago. We don't realize it still lives in us because it was encapsulated. It may last for years, even decades.

To encapsulate an experience of this kind is just what the brain does. But when a person's brain was balanced to begin with, it will tend to gravitate back to a state of homeostasis in time.

In the case of Jane, where there was an imbalance to begin with—as there is with many people—the unbalanced brain state tends to persist. The person is likely to begin experiencing minor physical problems. Perhaps they are more vulnerable to colds and flu. Since they are in a freeze state, they also find it difficult to be motivated. So when they most need to exercise, for example, they have no motivation to do so.

After going through two and half years in pain with their partner, perhaps they are now worried about taking care of their children. But this adds to their sense of abandonment and isolation, because they are so wrapped up in their children's lives that they are cutting themselves off from their own needs. Consequently, they start having a skewed view of reality. An issue comes up, and they look at it in a different way from the way they would usually see it. Their brain pattern is holding part of reality away from them.

When people experience this, they usually press on the gas pedal by tearing into a project. Then they lose interest as dissociation takes over again. So they tear into another project. The brain is attempting to balance itself, trying to get the sympathetic to take over from a heavy parasympathetic dominance. Still, the parasympathetic pattern persists because the brain doesn't know how to release it.

Sometimes people face a gastric problem when they experience persistent parasympathetic dominance. It may take the form of acid reflux or constipation. But if the dominance jumps to the sympathetic, diarrhea occurs. The two then alternate.

In females, this situation can trigger a hormonal change that results in night sweats and hot flashes. You may only be thirty-three, but you think you are going into menopause.

A Balanced Brain Makes for a Love of Life

When someone who competes in the martial arts loses their balance, they lose the contest.

Life itself is like that. We are going to get kicked at times. If our brain is off balance when life throws a kick at us, we are unable to move out of the way fast enough, which means we get hurt or knocked down. On the other hand, if our neural network is in balance, we have a natural instinct and ability to move in the manner called for by each situation.

Experiencing a meaningful life requires maintaining our balance. If we picture ourselves with the weight of the world on our shoulders, we feel we can hardly cope. With a balanced brain, we feel an "okayness" despite the fact we may be going through a difficult time. As a result, we find within ourselves the resilience to handle whatever life sends our way. We cope more effectively in even the most painful of circumstances.

For example, one female client reported, "Shortly after I trained my brain, my mother died. There were so many concerns to take care of, but I handled it all with ease. I was rational, competent, and didn't find myself becoming overwhelmed." It isn't that this woman didn't have a heavy load to bear; it's that the load didn't overwhelm her because her neural network was in balance.

When All Cylinders Are Firing Equally

Many of us have spent years functioning with an unbalanced brain. As a consequence, various aspects of our life have suffered.

For instance, people whose brain assessment shows a high parasympathetic function generally approach life from an academic, mechanical, or otherwise intellectual level, but they have difficulty feeling emotions.

Suppose such a person is asked in therapy, "What do you feel about what happened?" They may not be able to answer, or they may respond with what they *think* about the situation, which leads the therapist to ask again, "Yes, but what do you *feel* about what happened?"

This individual may be extremely competent in terms of executing tasks that need to be accomplished. They might even communicate on a sophisticated level. But it's all mentally oriented and not heart centered—and there is a world of difference between head and heart.

When a person can't feel their own passion, let alone the full range of emotions possible as a result of contact with others, they are dissociating to some degree. This is how we have created a world that's heavy on technology and consumerism but doesn't consider the effects on the environment that supports our existence. We are slowly doing ourselves in, but we can't feel it.

On the other hand, a strongly sympathetic-dominant person will likely be so "on guard" that they refuse to address the question of how they feel or just consider it irrelevant. Their defensive posture may sometimes be cracked open a little to expose a flood of emotions.

When we speak of balancing the brain, we are talking about allowing both the heart and the logic needed to execute a task to be present in appropriate amounts, given the particular situation. In a balanced brain, feeling and thought match each other, so that the end product of the person's actions is tailored to both a logical solution and one that everyone can feel good about.

In our present world situation, where global warming and the pollution of our environment with thousands of toxic chemicals have emerged as major threats to our wellness, the ability to rebalance our logic with feeling has become of critical importance.

Balance requires paying attention both to the concepts involved in performing a task and to the context in which the task is to be carried out. Equally, it requires attention to detail. For a balance to prevail, it's essential to be both logical and feeling.

When the brain is balanced, it is working in an integrated fashion, free of internal conflict between its regions. Each area of the brain is as active as it needs to be to support the activity of the other areas. It means we are firing on all cylinders, with the feeling and thinking aspects of our brain functioning harmoniously.

It's when we are firing on all cylinders that we can begin to catch a glimpse of our limitless potential. The brain is experiencing itself as optimized, which ramps up our ability to be what we were born to be. We are no longer restricted by the limited vision we have had of ourselves.

The following comment is representative of so many when their brain becomes balanced: "The calming effect of brain balancing has allowed me to access parts of my potential I didn't know existed. It enables me to push through issues that in the past would have stopped me cold." This person has gone on to have a successful career as a public speaker.

When our brain is functioning in an optimal manner, the waters seem to part for us. Because our brain is balanced, we see possibilities we might otherwise miss and pick up on opportunities others don't notice. This is because we think faster and more effectively, are more intuitive, feel more deeply, and put all our energy into acting creatively instead of reacting defensively. For an unbalanced brain, a lot of energy is continuously required to maintain composure and execute with some degree of effectiveness.

8

"Why Did I Do That?"

AT TIMES, ALL OF US FIND OURSELVES BEHAVING in ways that contradict our intelligence. It's not that we aren't good people or that we lack the desire to enrich our own life while enriching the lives of others. Generally, we want to do our best, and we can even be hard on ourselves when we fail. The problem is that behind much of our illogical behavior is an unbalanced brain, which prevents us from being the person we intuitively know ourselves to be.

Take anger, for instance. How often people say after losing their temper, "I didn't mean to blow up." They know it isn't helpful to erupt in anger, but it happens so quickly that it's usually over by the time they realize what they are doing. This is because the brain is locked into a pattern of behavior that's in the driver's seat. Consequently, when they get into certain situations, they are truly not free to do the right thing.

Dr. Bruce Lipton, a renowned cellular biologist and author of *The Biology of Belief,* explains that our cells are modified by the beliefs we hold and the actions we take. Cellular structure is actually altered by our behavior. For example, in the case of repeated outbursts of anger, the brain's neural network changes to the point it becomes *accustomed* to reacting in anger—even *addicted* to anger, because this has become the dominant brain pattern.

There was a time in my life when I felt extreme anger, to the point I behaved in ways that were self-destructive and hurtful to others. Generally, we don't do harmful things because we want to do them. We know they are harmful, but we can't seem to stop doing them. After each explosive episode was over, I invariably asked myself, "Why did I do that?" I knew my behavior was ridiculous. Then I compounded the situation with guilt. Despite all this, I continued this unsatisfying behavior.

Attempting personal change challenges each of us on many fronts, often on a daily basis. If we can't take in information and make it work in this present moment, then unfortunately we can't actually change. We can only consider change. We consider change every time we say a prayer. We consider change every time we sit in front of a psychotherapist or read a self-help book. I did all of these to try to help myself because I knew all-too-well I needed to change. I was aware of how my terrible rage was keeping people away from me, denying me the opportunity to love and be loved, for which I longed. I signed up for anger management classes, followed by extensive cognitive therapy. Nothing I tried enabled me to break the cycle of anger.

It took more than awareness of my anger and more than a desire to change for my behavior to actually change. For change to happen, the neural network of my brain had to undergo a transformation whereby existing pathways were dismantled and new links were forged so that brain flexibility was achieved.

Many of us use anger to relieve a parasympathetic dominance. If we get angry enough, we can certainly experience an increased flow of energy in the brain, but this lasts only as long as the rage lasts. For years psychologists suggested that people ought to indulge their anger in a safe environment to "relieve the pressure." The belief at the time was that people were bottling up their anger and needed to "let it out." To accomplish this release, people were invited to hit each other with rubber bats. Most of the couples who engaged in this process ended in bitter separations.

The trouble is, the brain goes right back to a parasympathetic dominance after the rage is over, which can be seen on brain scans. Now the person feels a lot worse. By indulging in rage, they temporarily sedate themselves, just as a person does with drugs or alcohol, and actually make their condition worse because the pattern becomes more deeply etched into the neural network. In due course psychologists began to realize that venting doesn't remove anger but exacerbates it.

Recapturing Our Natural State

Brain training takes a different approach to setting change in motion in our lives. Instead of encouraging us to resist the way we are, which leads to feeling as though we are at war with ourselves, training the brain begins with the recognition that the condition we seek to alter had a beneficial purpose at some point in the past.

This realization is crucial, because it enables us to befriend our present state rather than seeing it as our enemy. Then, instead of fighting with ourselves, we gently coax the brain into a state that's more appropriate for our present life.

Recall how Daniel, who we met in chapter one, grew up in an

almost permanent state of freeze, balled up emotionally like the fetus had balled up physically in the womb. This meant he was dissociated to some extent. Consequently, he wasn't very talkative. Although at home he would be loving, it was difficult for him to socialize outside the home where other children don't readily accept differences. To relieve his parasympathetic dominance, he gravitated to illegal substances. It wasn't that Daniel deliberately chose to make bad decisions, it was because he was being led by a brain pattern that kept him alive at one time.

When the parasympathetic is dominant, we can't "show up" as the person we really are. The only way this young man could break free of this pattern was either to use substances or to rage. Once he trained his brain, his parasympathetic dominance eased, the two sides of his autonomic nervous system began working harmoniously, and he didn't need illegal substances any longer.

Our negative behavior usually isn't a matter of there being something morally "wrong" with us. In each of us, inappropriate behavior is usually caused by outdated brain patterns that once served to protect us but that are no longer beneficial. Our brain was acting in response to a particular situation in the best way it thought possible at the time.

The change we seek can only become a reality when we recognize that what we are aiming for is actually our natural state. Because brain training returns us to this state, it provides us with a platform on which to make changes. We can put into action what we have longed to see happen—to be the strong, loving, healthy, and wise person we were born to be.

In other words, change isn't really change at all. It's not something we have to *do,* not something we have to *make happen*. Instead, it's simply allowing the essential person we are when our brain is balanced to emerge. It's a matter of allowing ourselves simply to *be.*

A Level Playing Field

Many of us have spent years trying to improve ourselves and the quality of our life. We have read books, watched informative talk shows, and even attended seminars on self-improvement. Some of us have also worked with personal coaches, pastoral counselors, and therapists. Although we may see improvement, often our progress is disappointingly slow and of limited success.

This is where brain training can be especially helpful, for it hands people a level playing field on which to reap the rewards of, say, psychotherapy. Whereas an individual may not have been able to get to the real issues before, with their brain balanced, they can allow themselves to *feel* and consequently *heal*.

Some believe that if we simply change our beliefs, we will overcome the things that hamper us. I certainly believe changing our beliefs can result in changes in our life. But there are often limits to our ability to make such changes, especially when our beliefs involve not only our external world but also how we feel about ourselves internally. Many of the beliefs we hold about ourselves don't readily yield to reason because they are ingrained.

We might liken the way patterns become etched into the brain to the effects of a minor auto accident versus a string of such accidents. When we have a minor collision, we usually recover from the shock quickly. But if we were to have a minor accident every day, this daily exposure would etch a deep pattern into our neural network. In such a case, it takes considerably longer for the brain to balance itself because the effects of the trauma have been so deeply and repeatedly inscribed in us.

Conventional approaches to entrenched imbalance have a poor success rate because it's extremely difficult to change a deeply etched pattern such as an inmate's beliefs about themselves and their fellow humans. To attempt to bring about significant change is akin to playing a board game on a table that's tilted to the point that anything you try to set on it rolls or slides off. Before you can begin the game, it's necessary to level the table. This is what brain training sets out to accomplish. It furnishes people with a level playing field on which to rebuild their life.

It's essential to realize a person can't even take in the information they need to rebuild their life until their brain is somewhat in balance. Only then can the brain receive the information that will bring change. Before a state of balance is achieved, the individual has little chance of accomplishing substantial change in their life. But level the playing field, and a change of belief about ourselves and others becomes realistic, leading to a changed life.

9

Is Your Brain Running in Overdrive?

IT'S OFTEN SAID THAT WE NEED to be "in the moment" if we wish to enjoy life to the full. The trouble is, most of us have difficulty being present in a manner appropriate for each moment. Hard as we try to be really present, we can often only manage twenty or thirty seconds without thoughts intruding.

Maybe some of us manage a minute. Except that, how do we know we lasted a minute? Did we look at our watch? "Well, I feel it was about that long," we say. The very fact we can say this means we were conscious of time and therefore not completely in the moment. As long as we are worried about coming out of the moment, we are not yet fully in the moment.

Picture yourself relaxing in a quiet, dimly lit room, with your feet up and your eyes closed. In such a condition, your brain receives comparatively little input, so your brainwaves should mirror a state of tranquility. It should be easy to be fully present, completely immersed in this relaxing moment.

In reality, when people are assessed in such a situation, many are found to be experiencing major brain activity. It's as if the individual were in a high-energy executive mode.

There needs to be congruence between what's happening in our external world and what's going on inside us. What would this look like? Low frequencies would dominate when we are expending low energy in a restful state. Medium frequencies would dominate when we are using medium energy, such as if we are thinking about something or watching television, but there's nothing intense going on at the time. High frequencies would dominate when we require a great deal of energy, such as for swinging a golf club, taking part in a debate, or working intently on a project.

Recall that we observed two Buddhist monks when formulating the template for brain training. When we assessed their levels of high frequencies during intense activity, their high frequencies were totally dominant. They were really "on," with razor-like attention. But when they closed their eyes and relaxed, their high frequencies plummeted, almost like flipping a switch. They had honed their ability to turn on and off. In the case of a person whose high frequencies are continually dominant, we are witnessing a severe imbalance. But in the person who can turn their high frequencies on and off as required, we are seeing the kind of brain flexibility that makes for optimal functioning.

Balancing the brain allows the neural network to reduce its energy output to where it is lower and slower when what we are doing doesn't require much energy. This not only enables us to handle routine matters more efficiently, it actually increases our capabilities because, instead of being lethargic as a result of continually running in overdrive, the brain is ready to perform at a high level when called upon to do so.

The Brain Under Siege

Young people everywhere are being diagnosed with attention deficit disorder. In the United States, eight percent of children ages four through seventeen are diagnosed with ADHD. Among adults, the percentage is between 2.9 and 4.4. However, it is believed that only a third to as much as a fifth of cases of ADHD are diagnosed.[2] This wasn't the case just a couple of generations ago. Why is attention deficit so prevalent today?

The input our brain receives has increased dramatically over the last fifty years. We are at a point where we are inundated with information and stimulation. Not only do thousands of bits of information flood into the brain from the natural world and our exchanges with other people every single second of a normal day, but to these we have added a vast input from technology. Think how much more challenging it is to drive in a modern city, with dense traffic, traffic signals and signs, pedestrians and cyclists, billboards everywhere, and all the hustle and bustle of city streets and storefronts, compared with riding a horse or driving a carriage down a peaceful country lane.

Some researchers suggest the input the modern brain receives may have risen as much as a thousand fold during the last half-century alone. So every second of every day, we are receiving a thousand times more input than were our grandparents. Even if this figure were only a hundredfold, it's still a huge increase in the input the brain has to cope with. It's not difficult to understand how a child's attention slips into deficit under such an onslaught.

When a child has ADHD, the prevailing wisdom is to medicate the brain with a stimulant. This increases the higher frequencies used for thinking, which overcomes the lower frequencies. However, increasing the higher frequencies with a stimulant causes the brain to become dependent on a chemical whenever it requires higher frequencies. Consequently, many who are medicated become addicted by the time they are eighteen.[3]

Alongside the vastly increased input the brain receives in a technological society, such a society also generates a great deal of busyness, which in itself can be a cause of imbalance. But it isn't only the way automobiles, trains, and planes allow us to rush around at a helter-skelter pace—and the telephone calls, emails, video conferences, and faxes that keep us interacting—that creates imbalance. We also wear ourselves out with all the pressure to perform that's placed on us in this kind of society. Instead of increasing our effectiveness, such pressure actually impairs our performance.

Take the matter of making decisions. In a culture in which we are so pressed for time, it's easy to fall into a habit of making decisions without the thorough attention each should receive. The trouble is that if we do this often, the low brain frequencies involved in such a decision take over as executive manager—a role they aren't equipped to fulfill. Pretty soon all our decisions circumvent logic and are executed from a "feel good" or "look good" mindset. Because this approach is hit-and-miss, it's hard to consistently make the best decisions this way.

Living in a technologically complex world, being busy almost all the time, and feeling pressure to perform lower the energy reservoirs of the brain. If there's little reserve of energy, a brain running at high speed will crash once its energy is depleted. This is similar to running so hard in a race that you run out of steam before the finish line.

Even when our brain is attempting to perform at its peak, its state of imbalance causes it to be far too busy to allow information to flow freely. In western society, it's likely that most who meditate aren't able to spend sufficient time in meditation to achieve the kind of balance that facilitates maximum flow of information. We don't become balanced enough because the chemical factory keeps pumping juices into the brain to generate activity—a function demanded by the brain activity itself, and hence a Catch 22.

When a person operates from this state, they don't sleep well. Consequently, when they awaken, they experience a slow start. They may have to drink coffee to get themselves going because coffee causes the blood vessels to constrict, which creates pressure. So now they start the pump again, running and running and running, until they crash again. If a person continually repeats this cycle, they eventually become so tightly wound that they have to reach for a glass of wine or some other drug to unwind.

Living under pressure causes no small number of us to feel continually on edge, which means we become easily angered. If we were to take an assessment of the brain of a person who feels this way, it would reveal they have a high-frequency dominance in a specific location compared with other frequencies in that area. A person with such a dominance is usually sufficiently volatile to have anger management problems. We say such a person has a potential violent streak in them and is quick on the trigger. Yet it isn't the high-frequency dominance that's the real danger, it's that the person's brain runs in this state all the time. When someone is at rest, their high frequencies ought not to be dominant.

When the brain isn't balanced and is firing too fast, it burns out sooner, which is eventually reflected in an impaired body. Also, with the brain so overactive almost all the time, a high degree of happiness is unlikely. Not impossible, but unlikely.

Take Charge of Your Time

A key aspect of success in the modern world is time management. On the surface, it seems like an easy subject. We are led to believe that all we need is a time management seminar or a seminar on efficiency in the workplace.

The most significant relationship any of us has is with time. Time management has to do with our entire approach to life, which is governed by the imbalance so many of us experience in our brain. Good time management is a matter of a balanced brain. When the brain becomes balanced, it allows us to reorient ourselves with respect to time.

In Native American culture, the idea of time management is to be present in the appropriate season. When it's harvest time, people in this culture want to harvest. When it's full moon, they might want to fish. Theirs is a seasonal approach, and they move with the seasons instead of resisting them. They are present with the flow of life, "in the moment" with nature. In western culture, we are rarely present with life's flow.

A second factor of native culture is that they evaluate time past to see what history has provided for them, what their ancestry has provided for them, and what their tradition has provided for them. They look first at the present, then second at the past. Only after this do they consider the future, and it's rarely a key concern since the seasons come on their own.

Native cultures don't fit well into Americanized culture, which looks first to the future, second to the past, and only third—and not easily— to the present.

Go to school to obtain credentials, get a good job, save your money, and get a good rate on it. We gear our lives around future expectations. This orientation towards the future puts a lot of pressure on us in terms of how we use our time now, in the present.

Consider how important learning institutions with their system of examinations have become to westerners. The entire way we prepare for a career is oriented around passing examinations. A lot of pressure builds up when a person's future is riding on a bar exam that will allow them to become an attorney, actuarial exams so they can become an insurance expert, accounting exams to become a CPA, or medical exams to become a physician. Candidates who take these examinations have all made an enormous investment of time and energy to reach this point. The pressure is tremendous, and they can't relieve the pressure because the system is designed around pressure.

Since our society doesn't spontaneously help us create balance when it comes to time management—since our society isn't designed to flow with the natural rhythms of time like Native American culture and doesn't facilitate being truly present in each moment of our existence—it's all the more important to be able to approach life with a balanced brain. For instance, a balanced brain can take much of the stress out of examinations. If individuals train their brain, their memory tends to improve, as do their verbal and writing skills, and they are more proficient when it comes to reasoning and making logical decisions.

Creating internal flow through brain training helps us to flow better, and therefore to be present, in a world that doesn't encourage flow.

Achieve Success Without Being Stressed Out

I once worked with a man who was preparing a doctoral thesis on mastery. I became interested in his research and interviewed a number of people considered to be masters, among them athletes, psychotherapists, and leaders in industry. Almost universally, none of these masters could describe how they do what they do. The fact is, they don't really know.

I asked one of them, "What about when you are not doing what you do well? How do you not do it well?"

He explained, "I'm usually distracted, uptight. I have other wants or needs at the moment. I'm not focused. I'm tense." We can't do something well if we're tense. We're using a lot of energy just to maintain this tense state—people actually clench their fists, arms, shoulders, or backs. In such a state, the brain isn't functioning optimally. The lack of flow in our performance reflects a lack of balanced brain energy flow.

The goal of training the brain is to enable it to see itself in an optimized state, and thus a kind of homeostasis is achieved. This is the brain's more natural state. In this state, it's simply a superb instrument, capable of propelling us to success in our career despite the obstacles we face. It enables us to function in far more helpful and productive ways than we are generally accustomed to.

For example, a twenty-seven-year-old female client writes, "I am a financial advisor, and so I need to help my clients make important financial decisions daily. I used to get bogged down with paperwork and preparing for meetings, always feeling stressed. I didn't know there was any other way to function in this kind of career. After a few sessions of brain training, I began noticing differences in the way I prepped for meetings. I found I was no longer second-guessing myself or over-analyzing situations. I was able to make my recommendations with confidence and poise, knowing that my clients were getting the best advice to allow them to meet their goals. This was a huge change from before—ask any of my colleagues! Though I'm viewed as one of the better advisors in the office, I lacked the confidence and conviction to convey this to my clients. As a result of these changes in my life, I attained my income and client acquisition goals for the entire year by the end of September."

In business, many people ply a lot of energy to get somewhere, but they don't give it quite enough and hence don't become a master. It's like bringing water to a boil. The temperature climbs fast at first. But when it reaches 205 degrees, it takes a tremendous amount of energy to go from 205 to 210, and a whole lot more to go to 211. But all we have at 211 is hot water. We have to take it one more degree before it boils.

Probably not one in a thousand takes it to the boiling point. People usually don't take this step because their fear intervenes. The fear sucks their energy out of them. We can actually see the dominance of fear in most of the lobes of the brain. So people give up long before they reach boiling point—the point of mastery and excellence. They tell themselves it's too hard. Or they start focusing on the problems they face, the information they don't know, the skills they lack, and the aspects of their life that aren't going well. Expending all this energy on negativity holds them back. But boiling point is just one degree beyond 211. All many of us need to take is just one more step, and this is what brain training can enable us to do.

When we train our brain, we lose none of our strengths—we simply discharge our brain static. This static consists of the fear that holds us back, the tension that keeps us from relaxing and allowing brain energy to flow freely, the mental fog that causes lack of clarity, the self-doubt that robs us of confidence, and the double-mindedness that splits our focus. As this static drops away, we become clear, intentional, purposeful. This is why the vast majority of people in sales who have trained their brain have increased their productivity dramatically. For instance, an advertising agency's account managers went from closing thirty percent of their pitches to closing sixty-five percent.

In the early days of brain training, I went to the office of an executive who had requested a demonstration. When I arrived, his administrative assistant said, "I don't think you should talk to him right now."

"Well, I'm already here and I've gone out of my way," I replied.

When I was shown into the executive's office, he looked terrible and certainly had no interest in talking to me. "I just lost the biggest deal I ever had!" he bemoaned.

"This is a perfect opportunity to train your brain," I explained. "Let me hook you up, and you can work on your computer without taking calls as your brain listens to itself. A state of anger and frustration may be the best time to see a major shift." Reluctantly, he agreed, and the training session revealed the severely unbalanced state of his brain. Within minutes of the training getting underway, his brainwaves altered dramatically. Although brain training couldn't undo the lost deal, he didn't have to remain in turmoil because of it. The loss no longer held power over his mood—and it no longer affected his administrative assistant, who sent us flowers!

Even when someone is gifted, some regions of the brain may be working more effectively than most of the neighborhoods. To put the individual's entire brain on a level playing field supports the exceptional areas so they can soar to greater heights in these specific areas. This particular executive went from one of the top ten achievers in Arizona to second in the nation in his field.

Though the corporate world doesn't yet consistently encourage people to become their very best, and still sometimes tries to take as much as it can without helping people see and reach for their full potential, there are companies such as Google that do an exquisite job of assisting their staff to reach for their potential. Such companies tend to be newer high-tech companies, along with the most successful of older companies, and they are leading the way into the world of the future. They create loyalty because of how they treat and remunerate their employees. Creating balance in the work environment may encourage brain balance and thus optimization of the workforce. I believe that someday companies will invite their employees to brain train, so that these employees can soar in their accomplishments both in the workplace and in their personal life.

Running Ahead of Our Evolution

Over eons of time, the brain has evolved filters that allow us to select which information from our environment will receive our attention. These filters enable us to concentrate on just a small portion of the available input, screening out the rest.

However, in our technological era, we suffer such an onslaught of information that it completely overwhelms the brain's filtering capability. Because these new forms of input have been thrust upon us almost overnight, we have had no opportunity to evolve more advanced filters. In other words, the evolution of society has moved faster than the evolution of the person.

As a result, we are at the point in our journey as a species where a growing number of people on the planet experience an imbalance early in life—an imbalance that's socially and technologically generated. Living in such a technologically complex society, we experience so much stress that our brain tends to run continually at a level of energy that's far too high, a level that should be reserved for moments requiring peak performance.

Although we have become accustomed to living in a constant state of stress from the extraneous input we receive in our kind of society, much of the time the brain doesn't need the throttle to be wide open. A balanced brain uses energy efficiently, which produces a harmonious result.

Harmony is desirable in most aspects of life. For example, think of brain energy in terms of musical notes. A note has a volume and it has a pitch. Notes of a higher pitch represent higher energy. For a tune to sound harmonious, it needs higher notes, middle notes, and lower notes. In most music, the tune is carried predominantly in the higher notes, whose volume tends to dominate the lower and middle notes. If a lower or middle note dominates when a higher note ought to dominate, the harmony is disrupted and the tune may be lost. For a brain to be in harmony, its energy must be balanced like a musical composition.

The brain's natural state is to be in homeostasis, and most of us are fortunate to begin life with a reasonably balanced brain. This state of homeostasis is the basis of health, happiness, creativity, and most importantly, love. It's the key to being able to be truly present in every aspect of our lives.

Using this platform of awareness, a person can establish lifestyle patterns that act as filters, thereby protecting the brain to some degree. For instance, a person whose brain is balanced—and who is therefore very present—will intuitively tend to seek out quiet times, peaceful situations, and the stillness of nature, all of which allow the brain a respite.

10

How a Brain Imbalance Often
Originates in Childhood

WHEN A BRAIN IS IN A STATE OF IMBALANCE, it's often the case that this arose early in life. Although the brain is a resilient instrument, in some ways it's also quite fragile, especially when we are young, before pathways in the neural network have become well established.

To understand the fragility of the infant brain, picture a teeter-totter with a small fulcrum. Because the fulcrum is tiny, the teeter-totter is easily tipped. The slightest movement can set it off.

For this reason, sometimes an imbalance originates before we were born, as in the case of Daniel in chapter one, or during the birthing experience. Birth is a traumatic event that, even when it happens in the most natural way possible, can trigger an imbal-ance. It's especially traumatic when there is a Caesarean section. Natural birth allows time for the brain to adjust to its entry into an entirely different kind of environment than it has previously known. After floating effortlessly in the warm environment of the womb, to be suddenly taken out of the mother instead of going through the gradual process of birth can be too much of a shock, putting the newborn brain into a state of fight or flight. Such an imbalance may cause the infant to see the world in a different way.

When the brain's frequencies rise to levels that are much higher than in a normal birth, a baby has a greater likelihood of having an overactive nervous system. By shifting into a pattern in which higher frequencies dominate in some areas, while lower frequencies dominate in others, the brain becomes focused on sensing what's going on around it but pays scant attention to thinking through details. What do we call a scenario in which there is too much activation in some areas, while lower frequencies dominate in others? Attention Deficit Hyperactivity Disorder. This is then compounded by the immense amount of information the brain has to deal with in our modern world, as we saw in the last chapter.

In the years following birth, children experience a variety of other physical threats that can trigger a brain imbalance. The most common of these is undoubtedly a bump on the head in early childhood.

Take the case of Michael, a forty-six-year-old man. As a child, he suffered a severe blow to his head as a result of a fall, yet he had no memory of the incident. Years later at a family reunion, he learned about the blow to his head from a relative who witnessed the event. The information proved to be a Godsend. For years Michael had been perplexed by a string of bad decisions that reflected poor judgment on his part. Little did he know that he had been functioning with an unbalanced brain throughout his life. Having heard about the many benefits of brain training, he wanted to experience it for himself. As his brain began to see itself in an optimized state, he discovered how profoundly the blow to his head had affected him. Training his brain set him on the road to a whole new understanding of himself and his capabilities.

The Role of Our Genes and Our Upbringing

Does our genetic heritage also play a role in how balanced our brain is? It can indeed, but often in a different way from what many of us have been led to believe by all the headlines about the effect of our genes on our health and well-being.

For example, the children of a parent who has knee problems tend to have more knee problems than the general population. Are their knee problems entirely a result of genetics? Or does the genetic map of the individual predispose the person to respond to life in a manner that adds to their vulnerability? In other words, their genetic map influences their diet, the activities in which they engage, what they believe about the state of their health, and a whole host of other environmental factors that exacerbate the underlying tendency. So their condition is partly genetic, partly learned from programming by their parents, and partly a matter of what they believe about themselves.

In similar fashion, the brain can become unbalanced as a result of the interplay of genetics and upbringing. Simply as a result of growing up, some of us have accumulated a serious imbalance in various parts of our brain. Our family experiences, together with our cultural and social environment, affected our brain in ways that created patterns we carry with us into adulthood. Sometimes these patterns are to our great detriment.

When a person has become accustomed to reacting in a certain manner in childhood, the neural network has literally been altered so that this behavior is automatic and even feels normal. When the person then finds themselves in an adult situation that mimics the environment that initially altered their cells, they will react in the manner to which they have become accustomed.

Emotional trauma, especially when experienced before an infant has formed a solid identity, can invoke an imbalance involving a parasympathetic dominance. For instance, if an infant is regularly faced with verbal or physical aggression, so that its environment feels unsafe, it has no means of either running away or standing up for itself—the fight-or-flight response. Its only defense is to freeze. In such circumstances, the infant brain establishes a pattern of blocking out the terror it feels by dissociating from the feeling.

Such is the case with Terri, an attractive woman in her late thirties who has worked her way up through the ranks to become a marketing manager in a large technology firm. In spite of the fact she is successful and independent, Terri is nine months into a relationship with Bradley, who on a daily basis tells her how unfit she is to be his girlfriend. He criticizes the way she walks, insisting she has a tendency to keep her hips too tight and doesn't swing them enough. When she speaks, he says she sounds unintelligible because she interjects words such as "like" into her explanations. When she eats, he complains she tends to gulp down her food instead of chewing it slowly. According to Bradley, she also skis without style, not making her turns sharply enough. Even her performance during sex is flawed. Despite all of this criticism, Terri isn't about to leave the relationship. Instead, she tries all the harder to please him. She's even now thinking of going to an ear, nose, and throat specialist because Bradley complains that when she is sleeping, she breathes too hard! This is the third relationship within two years in which Terri has selected a man who belittles her.

Someone close to Terri may wonder why, when Bradley puts her down, she consistently reacts by going into a submissive mode. Why doesn't she take action to change her situation? The fact is, Terri can't help but react this way. That she is forever walking on eggshells around men doesn't register in any way as abnormal with her because, while she was growing up, being put down was an everyday experience for her. Her neural network was so altered by an abusive home life that the derogatory treatment her partner dishes out actually feels deserved, perhaps even sought after. In such a situation, any information that may come to her on a cognitive level, suggesting that her reaction of simply submitting to abuse is misplaced, cannot be fully received because her neural network, which has long been conditioned to experience such a reaction as "normal," doesn't fully incorporate information to the contrary.

The Reason Children Play Violent Video Games

Another form of dissociation can be seen in the case of a five-year-old playing a violent video game. Shortly afterwards he strikes out at his brother, which results in a fight, followed by tears and being sent to his room. It's a common occurrence in many families. Often parents respond by threatening to take away the video game. If they actually follow through, there's usually hell to pay. The child pitches a fit, kicking and screaming, until the parent gives in and returns the game.

The debate about video games has tended to overlook why the child is drawn to violent games in the first place. It's widely assumed that it's the video game that's causing the child's violence. Surprisingly, brain scans reveal that most of the time it works the other way around. The video game is an attempt to resolve the aggression the child has stored up.

A child who immerses itself in violent video games tends to be dominant in either the parasympathetic or sympathetic nervous systems. *Imbalance* is the key word for such a child, in whom either the "brake" or the "gas pedal" is stuck in the on position. The child is carrying a great deal of suppressed aggression. It is suppressed because society insists that children not be allowed to feel their feelings as they arise. It's not considered "nice" or "polite" to even have such feelings, let alone express them. Playing violent video games becomes a way for the child to experience its thwarted aggression—and, of course, it sometimes spills out into how the child relates to other members of its family or its friends.

It's important to emphasize that the video games don't cause the violence. It's the suppressed aggression, built up from being made to live as a hostage to a brain imbalance so much of life. Playing video games is a way for the child to feel what it isn't permitted to feel in its everyday routine, and a way for it to offset the brain imbalance it experiences.

Violent video games act like an "upper." They are a drug of choice, selected in an attempt to counter an imbalance. The mind is attempting to restore a state of homeostasis, so it uses the video game to increase the activity of the sympathetic nervous system in the case of parasympathetic dominance, or simply as an energy outlet in the case of a sympathetic dominance. By stepping on the gas, it attempts to counter the firmly pressed brake pedal. Or, if the gas pedal is depressed already, it presses on it still harder, causing the sympathetic to go even faster so it will run out of gas, thereby restoring a temporary sense of balance from exhaustion.

Of course, the state of "balance" achieved by such an attempt at homeostasis isn't a healthy balance. The child is already high on either the parasympathetic or the sympathetic, and the games merely push it high on the opposite side. Now both sides are high, which creates a false sense of balance.

How stable is an automobile when you have the brake and the

gas pedal both pushed to the floor? It's no different in the case of the human brain. It takes almost nothing to disrupt such a false sense of balance and trigger an eruption. Why would someone erupt and even become violent? Such a response is an automatic reaction of the brain, which causes the individual to strike out to get free of the constraint of the imbalance. They take it and take it and take it, and then they explode. Picture a glass, filled to the brim. This represents the child filled with tension. One small drop will cause the glass to spill over—or cause the child to erupt.

If we were to ask a child in this state to hold out its hand before it plays the video game, we would see only a slight tremor. After playing the game for a while, the child's hand will be shaking. Of course, the child will claim to feel better because it truly believes it does. The effect is akin to that of drugs. It's a survival tool, just like drugs when adults self-medicate. This is why the first thing a child with an imbalance often wants to do when it arrives home from school is to get on the video game and stay there all evening, which often involves a continuous battle with its parents.

If a child's brain becomes balanced through brain training, the child's attitude toward video games may alter dramatically. This doesn't mean that a child with a balanced brain won't ever play violent video games. However, the reason for playing such games will be different, and the outcome will also be different. There will be nothing "driven" about the child's desire to play such a game. It won't be obsessed with the game.

By the time a child is four or five years old, it's possible to look at its brain in a noninvasive way and tell whether the child is likely to gravitate toward violent video games. It's possible to see the suppressed aggression, the imbalance of the autonomic nervous system.

In the case of a child who is addicted to violent video games, the child doesn't see itself as a real person in the game. This is how it is able to act out violence without having any sense of actually doing violence. The child can be so dissociated that it isn't emotionally connected to the characters in the game at all. It doesn't recognize that its attraction to the game is likely a reflection of an imbalance that creates a tendency to violence.

When a child dissociates, a violent video game becomes a means for the child to play an executive role, which is a feature of the sympathetic, while in a state of parasympathetic dominance. The child isn't really responsible—it's the brain imbalance that's at work. The same is the case with motorists who manifest road rage. Were we to look at their brains, we would see a similar pattern. In a state of total frustration, the individual is finally hitting the gas pedal with all their might.

11

Your Mind and Your Brain

Are Different

A MID-SIZED COMPANY WAS FACED with an extremely tight budget during an economic downturn, to the point that the CEO was tempted to make sweeping changes in the company.

This CEO was usually driven by anxiety at such times, which imparted a frantic tone to everything he did. Consequently, he didn't always think clearly, and certainly not creatively. During any crisis, this CEO usually expended much of his brain energy anxiously chewing over each detail of the crisis, which meant he wasted a great deal of time simply spinning his wheels. Already a workaholic, to combat the inefficiency created by his anxiety, he then drove himself all the harder. In due course, the additional stress this generated jeopardized his health. The pressure of living in a panicked state took down his immune system, first with a string of colds, then with a serious bout of the flu. Though he fought it, his body was forcing him to slow down, something for which he was not at all grateful.

In a sustained fight-or-flight mode like this, physical changes begin to occur at the cellular level in response to our disrupted body chemistry. In such a state, our own cells may then begin attacking us, which is what happens in the case of a cancer. Before long, the CEO discovered he had a pre-cancerous lesion in his stomach.

Just as many use drugs in self-destructive ways, this CEO had also been using a drug and had come to the verge of self-destructing, only his drug was acceptable to society: working himself to death. In an effort to strengthen his immune system, he embarked upon brain training, combining it with homeopathic medical treatment. Three months later, the lesion was gone.

When the latest financial crisis hit his company, the CEO, now operating from a more balanced brain, was able to recognize his initially panicked state, calm himself, and make decisions that weren't impulsive. As he pondered the company's situation and sought input from a variety of trusted advisers, there arose within him a clear sense that he needed to stand fast and ride out the recession.

The CEO was now basing his conclusions on something other than either his anxiety or sheer logic. As a result of training his brain, he was able to listen to what we call *intuition*.

What Is Intuition?

Sometimes people mistake "feel good" or "look good" decision-making for intuition, but real intuition isn't about flying by the seat of our pants. On the contrary, it arises when the brain is in harmony, whereby feelings and logic are both spontaneously incorporated into a decision. We are neither flying by the seat of our pants nor making a decision based purely on *logic*.

What is intuition? How does it work?

Intuition is a product of the *mind,* not the brain. There is a distinct difference between the mind and the brain. To understand intuition, we need to differentiate between them.

The brain is an information-gathering network that receives information from the senses and beyond. The information it stores is the basis on which any experience will be evaluated. However, as crucial as the brain is to the ability to experience a set of events, the brain isn't what gives us the sensation of having an experience. Anything that happens to us is nothing more than raw data until it's interpreted, and interpretation of the data is a function of the *mind.*

The interpretation of a set of events is based on an individual's past experiences and their personal values. This essentially occurs at the *subconscious* level of the mind. The conscious aspect of the mind then experiences the end result of this information processing.

Tor Norretranders, the Danish author of popular science books, has estimated that out of eleven million bits of information processed by the nervous system, only about seventy-five bits make up our conscious awareness.[4] For this reason, what one individual experiences in a given situation may be quite different from the experience of another person in the identical situation. For instance, on a rollercoaster or skydiving, one may be experiencing the thrill of a lifetime, while the other is petrified. In sex, one may be experiencing pleasure, the other a sense of violation. It all depends on which brain pattern the mind uses to interpret a particular experience.

The brain is a network that supports the mind in its task of processing the information contained in the network. In this sense, the brain is similar to a computer program such as a spreadsheet. Let's say the spreadsheet is set up to calculate the taxes you owe. You list your income in one column of the spreadsheet, while in another column you list your expenses. The spreadsheet calculates the exact amount of your revenue, subtracts expenses, which gives you your profit, then tells you the taxes you owe. The calculation in this example is a form of information processing.

When you were a child running around the yard having fun, you didn't have to worry about taxes. Then came the day you were sufficiently grown up to begin earning, and all at once you were required to pay taxes. At first, figuring the tax was straightforward because you had simple earnings with few expenses. You just paid a percentage of your income. But as your ability to earn became more sophisticated, figuring your taxes required keeping a considerable amount of data for processing in a spreadsheet. At this point, you likely required a tax accountant to run the calculations for you. In the case of the brain, as an individual accumulates more and more information to be processed, the neural network expands to handle the increase.

The brain is a network running a program that allows information to be stored and shared. It works much like active memory in a computer. The more functional memory we develop by increasing the complexity of the neural network, the more data we can process. The information we garner from the five senses supports the mind, feeding it the data it needs to perform its duties as the value-based command center for the body.

Although the brain is an extremely complicated network, it's still just a network. To return to the analogy of the brain as a computer and the computer program as the brain's patterns, no matter how valuable the computer and its programs may be to us, it is simply a tool. Similarly, the brain is a tool—it isn't who we essentially *are*. The difference in the case of the brain is that it isn't optional like a computer. The mind and brain are interdependent and we cannot *be* who we are without the brain. In fact, the degree to which our brain works well determines the degree to which we are able to derive fulfillment from our experience and express ourselves through a rich participation in life.

The mind cannot function effectively without a balanced brain. We have already noted that a brain in optimal condition is balanced between the left and right sides, as well as from front to back. Additionally, in a fully balanced brain, the energy in each of the lobes is in harmony. In other words, the brain's energy is optimized.

We might liken a balanced brain to instruments playing in an orchestra. Not only do the individual instruments play in harmony within their own section of the orchestra, their volume is balanced and they follow a common rhythm. Each of the different sections of the orchestra also plays in the same key and maintains a balanced volume. In the case of the brain, the more finely tuned the network is—in other words, if the connections in the neural network are well made and the network is flowing smoothly—the more readily information stored in the brain is available for the mind to process whenever such data is required.

The mind is a development of a much higher order than the brain. The mind functions more like a series of algorithms, which connect information to form meaningful patterns—much like the early algorithms I helped develop when I was with Net Perceptions connected the customers of a bookstore like Amazon to other books they might enjoy. The power of the mind increases as its algorithms multiply, enabling us to derive greater meaning from the information our senses take in.

Let me try to put all of this a little more clearly. A purposeful life can't be achieved simply by accumulating information, which is strictly a function of the neural networks of the brain. The real issue is what we do with this information. The brain provides the data, but it's the mind that processes the information and puts the data to work in a meaningful way. The mind creates information value. The degree of fulfillment a person is able to enjoy is proportionate to the information they possess coupled with their ability to use this information effectively. In some cultures, they call the ability to use information effectively the attainment of *wisdom*.

How Your Brain Works

The brain and the mind are not the same thing. But though they are separate, they are interdependent. What the mind *is* becomes apparent when we understand what the brain *does*.

The brain is a network that performs computations. In this sense, the brain is akin to a computer network. The mind requires a brain that functions reasonably well, yet it is in no sense the equivalent of the brain or the interactions of the brain's various neighborhoods. The mind is the equivalent of the information processing carried out by the brain.

The mind is what enables us to care about things, furnishing us with goals, direction, values, and meaning. It's this ability to care about things—to value some things above others—that brings us both satisfaction and a sense of purpose.

How the brain learns, stores, and recalls what it learns is a complex process—far more complex than how a computer archives information.

The information used by the mind is actually stored in multiple places in the brain. For this to happen, a memory must be broken into many pieces, which are sorted according to the particular type of information involved. This is because any given memory of an event consists of a variety of distinct features. Some of the data concerns the overall picture of the event—the context. Other aspects relate to the details of what happened. Smells, taste, touch, sight, and sound are all different aspects of a memory, each of them related to different compartments of the brain's neural network. Added to these are the feelings associated with the event. These are manufactured by the brain's chemical factory. All these different types of information that make up a particular memory are stored throughout the brain.

How the brain breaks information down into its various components for storage in different parts of the network can be compared to sending an email. As we type, our email appears in the form of a page. But when we press "send," the information in the email can be separated into a host of electrical impulses, which is the mode of transmission over the web. In other words, our email is literally segmented.

It's necessary to break up an email because, at the same moment we may be sending an email, millions of other computer users are also sending emails, and there is only so much bandwidth through which data can travel. To facilitate the flow, the channels are packed as tightly as possible. To accomplish this, the bits and pieces of each email are separated out and combined with similar bits and pieces of other emails. This allows for the maximum utilization of the channels of transmission. The network switches the bits and pieces of an email into whichever channels are available to speed it on its way. Part of your email may be in one piece, and another part stuffed up against someone else's email to keep the flow up. Only at the end of its journey are the various parts of the email brought back together to form a cohesive message. All of this usually happens in milliseconds.[5]

How do the different bits of an email know where to go on the network? The answer is that each bit is coded. How this works can be seen from a visit to the drive-in window of a bank. We place a deposit in a canister so it can be sent to the teller. Each of the cans from several different drive-in windows ultimately pass through the same delivery tubes, then are separated out to arrive at different tellers. How does a canister know to zip back to a particular teller? Each can has a specific signature attached to it so that the system knows where to take it. Similarly, in the case of an email, a code attached to each of its parts tells it where to go so it can be reassembled on the recipient's computer screen.

When the Neural Network Is Impaired

In early 2008, a key communications cable carrying the worldwide web was severed on the seabed of the Mediterranean. The break caused an enormous disruption of the internet, necessitating the rerouting of much information. Overall, the global web still functioned, though less efficiently—and, in some areas of the world, communication was drastically reduced.

A similar situation can arise in the brain. If it develops a less than optimal pattern for processing information—a pattern that originates in an experience in which it had to act defensively to keep itself alive—it functions much the same as the worldwide web with a major cable cut. If the part of the brain affected happens to support memory, the memory will be affected. If the part affected supports thinking, then the individual's ability to think clearly will be impaired.

As long as the brain is functioning according to an outdated pattern, information the mind has can't readily impact the neural network. Even if the individual has an experience that helps the brain override the earlier pattern, this earlier pattern will still deplete energy that would otherwise be better used by an optimized brain.

For instance, one man discovered shortly after he turned sixty that, as a child, he had suffered a concussion that resulted in almost the whole of his right brain being impaired. Over the years, positive experiences had stimulated his left brain to take on many of the right brain's functions. But there was a cost. His brain was using three times the energy of a balanced brain, which meant he frequently found himself exhausted.

Because the brain is the tool the mind uses to process information, we cannot process any form of information unless the neural network is relatively functional. To the degree that the brain is damaged and its network impaired, the mind's ability to both garner information from the senses and also express itself through the senses will be limited. When the brain is optimized through brain training, memory and thinking are likely to improve.

In the case of a balanced brain, what the mind learns can have a profound effect on the brain. Just as events can alter the structure of the brain, so also can the mind alter the structure of the brain. It can do this because it has the ability to integrate information in a manner appropriate for any given situation. Instead of having to think out answers to situations that present themselves to us, which takes time, the mind has the ability to process the information in the neural network in a way that enables it to *intuit* the solution we seek.

Intuition Is Based on What We Value

Intuition is the ability to determine, almost in a flash, what we value in any given situation. It's a function of the mind, but it only works accurately when the brain is in a state of homeostasis.

In a nutshell, intuition says, "This is what I want!" It reaches its decision quite apart from thought. Information that is intuited is simply received and not a result of processing.

The *brain* has no interest in values. As we have seen, its primary purpose is to keep us alive. In and of itself, it doesn't care what we value or don't value. How valuable is a particular piece of information to us as an individual? How valuable is it to the people in our life or to the world in general? When is it most valuable? How might we best apply it? To ascertain the value of information is the basic work of the *mind*. As an information processor, it evaluates everything in terms of value.

Value is something each of us measures according to our particular genetic heritage, our upbringing, our personal experience, our unique personality, and many other factors. In other words, assigning value to something is a highly subjective art that depends on the specific brain patterns each of us has developed. It's for this reason that we are all so different—that we have different interests, different skills, and value different things. Our neural networks are all quite unique.

When the human brain is unbalanced, it tends to distort the value of information. To put this in tribal terms, if your tribe identifies everyone in the tribe as human and everyone beyond the confines of your tribe as subhuman—in the manner that Europeans regarded the indigenous peoples as subhuman when they explored the continent of Africa—you will tend to regard such people as having no intrinsic value of their own. This means that their only value is their value to you, which allows you to use them as a resource. You may kill them if they obstruct your goals, and you may enslave them to accomplish your purposes. This mentality was once the way the whole world thought. Even today, many tribal conflicts in various parts of the world are based on the same distorted value system.

This tribal mentality is often evident in religion, especially the more sectarian forms of religion. A person joins a sect and begins to think of themselves as part of the "tribe," or what they might term more benignly their "church family." They identify with the teachings of the group and with the leader. They adhere to the particular practices of the group. Years later, an individual may leave the community. When they look back, they are astounded at how they gave up their freedom, surrendered their mind, and turned over their worldly goods to the sect. How does this happen?

When someone's neural network is unbalanced, they are ripe for conquest by a belief system they feel is going to bring about homeostasis. The brain craves homeostasis. So when the neural network is in a condition of severe disharmony, the person will be drawn toward extreme beliefs and practices that promise a small amount of relief from the imbalance.

The rise of Nazism and Stalinism are classic examples of how unbalanced brains gravitate toward a degree of zealotry that, when viewed from the perspective of a more balanced mind, is hard to fathom. Once the person is ensnared, they find themselves in a loop. They have accepted certain information because their brain wanted to feel the "balance" that comes from homeostasis, and now they are incapable of thinking outside the loop. They believe what they believe because they are a member of the tribe, and they are a member of the tribe because they believe what the tribe believes. In other words, imbalance led to certain beliefs being fed into the network, and from this point on anything that contradicts those beliefs and threatens to disturb the artificial homeostasis that's been established is automatically rejected. It matters not that the beliefs may be entirely erroneous; it's the feeling of homeostasis and perceived safety such beliefs provide that counts. It's this false sense of harmony that defines value for the individual.

When the brain is brought into a true state of balance and harmony, it can't be easily pulled into a destructive tribal mentality any longer. Why is this? When the brain is balanced, our intuition comes into play to a greater degree. Once our intuition is active, we have the ability to evaluate information with a detection device that is parallel in power to our value system. We can sense when something is "off."

Our information processor functions to make the value of information clear, and this value is always proportionate to the level of good the value represents. In other words, it evaluates information according to the best thing for each of us as individuals, coupled with a concern for the greater good. The wise path will always lead to our well-being and the well-being of others. It will further our evolution, growth, health, and ability to be helpful. Any time information doesn't take us in this direction, a person whose brain is balanced will intuitively question the value of the information regardless of the apparent "logic" thrown at them.

The only reliable value system is that which comes from a combination of intuition, experience, and logic. As long as our values are based only on thinking or emotion, they are subject to the limitations of the tribe that imparted these brain patterns to us. Until we actually begin seeing ourselves—our essence, beneath the layers of thought and emotional reactivity—we cannot know what's of real value.

If our life experience is based only on the norms of the tribe, our view of the world can be terribly distorted. This is why connecting with our intuition is crucial. It allows us to process information in a more holistic context so that we gain the perspective of balance. Intuition safeguards us by showing us the big picture and how to apply it to life's puzzles.

When we bring a balanced worldview to the tribe, and this is augmented by the balanced worldview of other members of the tribe, ultimately the entire tribe tends toward a healthy balance.

12

Living Consciously

A PARTICULAR EXECUTIVE was a highly competitive individual to whom getting ahead of others meant everything. Because of the pressure he put on himself throughout the workday, by the time he left the office for his commute, he was extremely high strung. The drive home became a way to take out his tension on other drivers. He had a fast car and delighted in speeding whenever he could.

Each evening, at a particular point in his commute, this executive came up over a rise where two highways merged into six lanes of solid traffic. At this juncture in his journey, the competitive spirit that had driven him all day reached fever pitch. Getting ahead of any vehicle in front of him became a goal. He drove dangerously, cutting in and out, weaving his way past one car after another.

Every time the executive could pass another driver, he saw it as a victory, regardless of the angry gestures and verbal insults yelled out of open windows by other drivers. The executive didn't care how many people he upset.

By the time this man arrived home each evening, he was totally uptight from having driven like a maniac. To calm himself, he used alcohol—and, as time passed, he required an increasing quantity to take the edge off. A person who is bouncing off the ceiling can't turn off, can't get to sleep readily, which is why so many use alcohol or drugs to put themselves to sleep, as did this man. Not only was he burning himself out, his relationship with his wife was suffering because he was either too busy or too inebriated to relate to her meaningfully.

When this man embarked on the task of balancing his brain, it was with the idea it would help his golf game. But after only six training sessions, he remarked, "Last night I came up over the rise. The usual six lanes of congestion lay ahead of me. But instead of getting upset as I usually do, I suddenly saw myself as if I were part of a caterpillar along with the other cars, and we were all moving through the landscape together."

The man had caught a glimpse of what happens when we experience a routine event from a state of consciousness in which we recognize we are all part of a single universal reality. By becoming aware of himself as part of the whole, instead of seeing himself in competition with the whole, his need to get ahead of others diminished and a peace replaced his competitive frenzy.

Now when he arrives home, he doesn't need alcohol to calm himself down because he is already relaxed. Instead of anaesthetizing himself, he is ready to spend quality time with his wife. In fact, they have taken up a hobby together.

Because the executive is approaching life from a higher consciousness, he finds people gravitating to him, seeking his friendship, even when he makes no attempt to draw them to himself.

They come simply because his contentment is infectious. As a result, he and his wife have embarked on a new chapter in their lives—one of expansion, creativity, and helpfulness.

At some point, going through all that trauma every evening would have taken a toll on this man if he hadn't trained his brain. Driving in a fight-or-flight state would likely have resulted in an accident in which he might have killed an innocent motorist, then had to deal with shame and guilt for the rest of his life, and perhaps even prison. Or he might have killed himself. There was also a serious risk that using increasing quantities of alcohol would lead to him becoming addicted to the very substance that was calming him down. A heart attack or other health risks could also have been on the horizon.

This executive's risky lifestyle was based on the way he understood value, which came from the unbalanced way in which his brain functioned. Getting ahead of everyone, which he valued above all else, wasn't based on who he really is. The insane person behind the wheel who saw himself in competition with everyone wasn't the real person at all. His essence knew him to be part of a universal whole, but he wasn't able to see this until he began training his brain. His neural pathways were too distorted to process information available to him from this level of consciousness.

The End of Fear, Competition, Strife

Humans are mostly driven by fear of each other instead of by a sense of being part of an integrated whole. This is what triggers the terrible wars and genocide that occur with seeming regularity on our planet.

We can see this from pre-World War II Germany. There was extreme inflation, resulting in widespread poverty and hunger, with breadlines everywhere. When people are worried they won't be able to eat, fear replaces reason. So when Hitler expounded his simplistic solutions to Germany's problems, it was almost inevitable the masses would rally around him. He knew how to appeal to people whose brain networks were traumatized. This led the German nation down a path of severe imbalance, resulting in millions of our fellow humans losing their lives.

On a lesser scale, fear grips people when there are attacks by terrorists. In so many places in the world today, people feel vulnerable on their own soil. When such attacks happen, the media remind people of what has happened every minute of every hour of every day, until individuals who were nowhere near the attack are traumatized and fearful. As a consequence, a whole group of people's neural networks enter into a collective imbalance.

Fear causes us to be suspicious, defensive, competitive, and combative. At the very time when accurate information processing is most needed because it's critical to assessing how our values should be applied in a situation in which we are under threat, an imbalance hijacks our neural network. This causes us to feel alienated from both our own essence and that of others. When this happens, we make a mess of our lives—and a mess of our world.

The risks that accompany an imbalance in the neural network are even more serious when an entire nation is driven by such brain patterns. We live in an era when a reactionary brain pattern is especially dangerous because of the risk of rogue nations or terrorists getting their hands on nuclear or chemical weapons. When a reactionary brain pattern is in charge on this scale, individuals become a danger not only to themselves and to those in their immediate vicinity, but also to our whole species.

Fear is a movement away from homeostasis. Homeostasis is the condition of love and connectedness, and you can see it in a brain pattern. The degree to which a person bases their decisions on fear is measurable in a brain assessment, as is the degree to which the person makes decisions based in love.

As we recognize our connectedness, what drives us changes. No longer does fear dominate the decision process. When the brain is in a state of homeostasis, fear and defensiveness don't take us over so easily. This is when love can happen—a love of self, a love of others, and a love of life.

Part of Everything, and Everything Part of Us

Each of us is one of more than six billion people who inhabit this planet. When we think of ourselves in this way, we feel small. When we look at the size of this planet compared with the size of our solar system, we feel even smaller. If we then consider that our solar system is but one speck in a vast universe, we realize we are infinitesimally small. Compared with the number of grains of sand on every beach of every continent of the world, we don't even amount to a single grain of sand.

Quite apart from our smallness in light of the size of the universe, all of us have at times had the experience of feeling small in everyday life. Beginning with being a child, most of us at one time or another felt intimidated by other children and wished we were bigger. We fantasized that if we were the biggest person on the playground, no one would mess with us. We would never have to worry about someone taking our sandwich at lunchtime or making fun of us.

In view of our seeming smallness, how are we to think about ourselves? When we allow ourselves to think beyond ourselves, we entertain questions about what's valuable in our life. We want to

122 LIMITLESS YOU

know: How should I measure my value? What gives my life significance besides possessions? What makes me happy, contented, and secure? What makes me feel good about myself? These are the questions the competitive executive finally asked himself. The issue raised by such questions is how we perceive ourselves in the world.

Seen from the point of view of our size, a single human life appears all but insignificant. But our significance has nothing to do with our size. The reality is, we each participate in the most significant entity there is in the universe—the consciousness out of which the cosmos itself arises.

As the executive came to see in the imagery of the caterpillar crawling through the hills, we are not discrete, disconnected individuals struggling to survive, trying to "make it." Though the view so many of us have of ourselves as separate, independent entities seemed logical when viewed through the lens furnished by Newtonian physics, from a quantum standpoint this view of ourselves has been shown to be fundamentally flawed. We may appear to be separate entities, but in reality we are each an embodiment of an interconnected, single web of existence.

Our significance rests in something even more profound than the fact we are each a manifestation of what one scientist has called "the whole shebang." We are not just products of the universe, we are part of the field of *being* out of which the universe has sprung, and the essence of this field is consciousness.

An Informational Universe

Knowing ourselves to be one with the whole of reality not only gives us a sense of security, it also provides us with a source of information that isn't accessible through the five senses. This is especially important when, both as individuals and as a world, we face difficulties for which we have no answers.

Science has shown us that a far greater pool of information exists outside of the particles that make up matter than is contained in the particles themselves. The universe is an informational field, of which our individual consciousness is a manifestation.

Because we are linked with the entire cosmos, part and parcel of the whole, the information stored in the entire vast field of existence is available to us if we know how to tune into it. The information isn't in the mind or the brain, it's in the quantum soup of which the cosmos is composed.

We have tended to think of consciousness as something generated in the brain. From a quantum worldview, it's possible that consciousness arises from a very difference source—that there exists around us a field of consciousness, of which our individual consciousness is simply a focused expression. In other words, it's as if we were each a receiver and a transmitter, tapping into this field of consciousness and then broadcasting it to the world around us on our unique frequency. The mind functions as the information processor for our particular expression of this universal field. If this is the case, in order to increase our consciousness, one of the things we need to do is to balance our brain so that information can flow more effectively.

It's because we have been schooled in the Newtonian worldview that we tend to think of consciousness as arising in our individual brains, instead of seeing it as a universal field that seeks to express itself through us. Though the information of the quantum field is beyond us, we can pick it up and process it in the brain if we know how to tune into it. This is how people we call seers—people we think of as psychic—are able to pick up information. It's also why their insights are often only partially accurate. They are intuiting something from the field of consciousness, but their ability to access it is fragmentary, and hence their conclusions can be somewhat hit and miss.

Our ability to tap into the information field that lies outside us also explains a curious phenomenon seen in the work of Nobel Prize winners. Many of these brilliant individuals have had the experience of other experts in different parts of the world working on the identical discovery at the same time, despite the fact none of them knew of each other's research. This is no coincidence, for it has happened repeatedly. Invariably, when a new field of discovery emerges, we find someone else in a different part of the world working on the same discovery. The implication is that when a breakthrough occurs, it's because we have attained a level of evolution at which there is a readiness for the new information to come into play.

The part our physical brain supplies in this equation is the antenna to pick up the information available to us in this quantum dimension of consciousness. It appears that the input comes through receptors in the back of the brain. These receptors are able to receive information from beyond the confines of our senses. But whether information comes through the five senses or from beyond us directly to the mind, it's all processed in the brain.

We think of certain individuals as masters in a particular field of endeavor. The person might be a scientist, physician, baseball player, writer, or musician. Such individuals are masters not simply because of their natural ability, although this is of course an essential part of the package. They are masters because they have honed their ability to receive information, developed the necessary channels for this information to go immediately to their frontal lobes for execution, and established a neural network that allows for the effective carrying out of decisions. They are also masters because they have created efficient patterns for their brain to work on tasks related to their field.

We can see how fast the field of consciousness is capable of informing our intuition in the case of a baseball player who is a master of his art. Up against a really fast pitcher, there simply isn't time for him to actually see the ball, determine where the pitch will be over the plate, and then decide whether he should swing at it. It's physically impossible to see it and cognitively process the information. But a really good hitter is able to "see" it in a different way. He *feels* it, intuits it.

An experienced player knows when the ball is going to come over in the strike zone. How does he know? Since he's done it countless times, he has a pool of data to draw from. His consciousness surveys this information, which is stored in the brain's network, then sends an intuitive decision from the mind back to the brain for execution. This all happens in far less than a second. His mind asks: Is this ball going to be in the strike zone? Will I swing at it? If so, how hard will I swing, and how fast? Which part of my anatomy do I need to move to start the swing? All of these questions are asked and answered in a flash.

How does the brain work to clarify all the information we receive so rapidly that it's almost instantaneous? It happens in a dimension that's beyond our thinking ability—the dimension of consciousness.

Consciousness is pre-thought. It's a "knowing" that doesn't require thought, but that powers intuition, moving at the speed of light. But consciousness isn't the antithesis of thought, it simply doesn't run on thought. When necessary, it generates constructive, helpful thoughts to enable us to carry out what we intuit.

A balanced brain allows the "knowing" that resides in the field of consciousness to move into our awareness, where it can inform us of the accuracy or inaccuracy of information. This "knowing" isn't information per se. It's an intuitive response to the information we receive from other sources. It's what Jesus had in mind when he said the spirit within us would "teach us all things" we would need to know. There is nothing religious about this statement. On the contrary, Jesus was a master who understood the power of living from the intuition that flows from the field of consciousness, and he invited us to join him in this grand enterprise.

The Enlightened Night of the Soul

We tend to associate the coming of nighttime with darkness, and we use the term darkness metaphorically to refer to ignorance. However, while we speak of "the dark night of the soul" as a time of spiritual desolation, it's also the case that with nightfall there frequently comes illumination.

Consider some of the great creative geniuses who have had such an impact on our lives—people like Edison and Alexander Graham Bell. Such individuals reported that they had ideas come to them from somewhere seemingly beyond them. Many of them mention this happening when they were almost in a sleep state, but not quite. Why is insight of this nature associated with nighttime?

If we go to a busy beach toward the end of the day, when the tide has been out for several hours and the crowd has left, there are so many footprints running in different directions that it's impossible to follow a particular trail. But then the tide comes in during the night and the waves wash away the footprints, leaving the beach pristine, with not a trace of human activity upon it. If we now walk along the beach, the footprints we leave behind are so clearly defined that anyone can follow them.

Sleep has a similar effect on the busy neural pathways of the brain. When we are on the verge of sleep, the busyness of the brain recedes. As the network becomes quieter, it's more receptive to information from the field of consciousness. When we are in a close-to-sleep state—whether at bedtime, during the night, or toward morning—frequencies from the back of the brain, where we are in touch with universal consciousness, are able to move forward more readily. Because the brain is quiet, there's less interference to block their path. In such a tranquil state, information from the field of consciousness is more apt to reach our executive manager, which resides in our frontal lobes. This is how a sudden intuition comes to us at such moments.

What if we were to balance our brain so finely, we could readily access the vast pool of information beyond ourselves? If we could work from both the intuitive side of our brain and the logical side simultaneously, we could receive outside information in a continuous stream. This ability would place us in a perpetual mode of creativity. At that point, we would be linked with everything that exists.

I believe that to become enlightened isn't a "spiritual" happening of the kind so many imagine. It's simply to begin living from a much different principle from how most of society functions. Instead of life being a continual struggle, we realize we aren't separate individuals each trying to make it from day to day. Rather, we are all intrinsically connected to the whole, and therefore part of something much greater than ourselves.

We are invited to live in the realization that we are each an important part of consciousness itself. Becoming aware of this enables us to receive information—guidance—from the universal consciousness that is our essence. This is the experience of enlightenment.

Consciousness Is Power

The way to increase our power is to increase our awareness of our oneness with everyone and everything. If we really knew we are intrinsic to the greatest reality there is, it would so empower us, so boost our confidence, we would exude greatness. If we could all realize we are part of the whole, it could eliminate conflict. To have this sort of awareness would give us the kind of power that can end wars forever. If the divine encompasses everything, and we are one with the divine, then it follows that if the divine is for us, as one ancient writer put it, who can be against us?

When we talk about increasing our consciousness, we are talking about bringing a direction to the information processing that takes place in our brain under the command of the mind. The more our consciousness expands, the more we find ourselves with a sense of direction. The more honed our direction becomes, the more we are integrated into the whole, and the greater our sense of our value. In fact, I believe that when the power of higher consciousness begins directing brain patterns, it creates a snowball effect for well-being.

Consciousness invites us to recognize *being* as the source of all truly effective *doing*. Especially in America, though also in the West in general, as I mentioned earlier, we tend to be humans *doing* and not humans *being*. Because we don't know what being is, we lack a sense of feeling "okay" without having to perform in some way. In this culture, our value is usually based on what we do, what we've accomplished, or how much money we make. In fact, these days our value is almost wholly based on externals rather than on how much we have grown in consciousness and contributed to the advancement of our fellow humans.

Integrity is the barometer of consciousness, and it requires consistency of intention. But the intention we wield isn't narcissistic—

it doesn't revolve around seeking to bolster our sense of "okayness" by means of material things or accomplishments. Rather, intention that has integrity is based on a vision of our collective value and how we see ourselves within this collective value.

When the brain is balanced so that the information processor—the mind—can function effectively, what we are doing is combining and integrating the sphere of science and the spheres of value, ethics, and spirituality. This merger is where pure magic happens.

Quantum physics has shown us that the universe is a single reality manifesting as countless forms. We may be infinitesimal in terms of the vastness of the universe, but we could not be more important. In us the cosmos is aware of itself. In and through us, the creation is able to observe and enjoy itself.

The cure for feeling small is to become conscious of our intrinsic oneness with the universal reality that has birthed everything. When we are aware of ourselves as part of the infinite source, we realize we are essential to the universe's ability to be what it is intended to be.

Once we realize this—once we really *get it*—we experience a profound sense of groundedness, which means we have no reason to feel small ever again. Each day, in all the many facets of our lives, we experience a connectedness instead of the false sense of separateness that leads to competition, defensiveness, and feelings of smallness and inadequacy. Recognizing ourselves as part of the whole, our life has integrity within this whole. We are one with our fellow humans, one with the world of nature, one with the galaxies—indeed, one with the entire cosmos.

We are big people because we are each part of a truly "big deal."

Coming up over the rise and seeing the lanes of cars ahead of us, we understand ourselves as part of the whole instead of being in competition with the whole. That's magic. That's the kind of quality of life that produces real fulfillment.

13

An Antidote to Depression

LOOKING AT THE BRAIN ASSESSMENT of a woman who had been a partner in a large financial institution, I could tell she was the kind of person who is driven. "You are a strong type A personality," I remarked.

"Very," she admitted. "I want things done, and I want them done a certain way."

"Did you come from a family in which at least one parent was exceedingly critical?" I asked.

"I could never do enough," she affirmed.

"Were you the responsible one in the family?"

"I was the oldest and I took care of all my siblings."

"You have a strong defense, which means you don't crumble easily. Your drive is your defense, right?"

"You got it. I'm the go-to gal. If there's a crisis, everyone comes to me because they know I can cope."

"But your brain map tells me you have an underlying depression because carrying all this responsibility has worn you down."

"That's exactly right!" she exclaimed. "I've been on antidepressants for ten years."

"The ongoing depression and treatments are part of the reason your extremities move much of the time. You don't have a tremor, but you demonstrate a great deal of involuntary movement."

When such symptoms as involuntary movement occur in a person, it's because there's a conflict between different parts of the brain. One part is in a mode geared to taking information in, whereas another is attempting to send information to the body to initiate action.

How does what's happening in the brain show in the body's extremities? An example is when our fingers happen to get too close to a hot stove. As the heat begins to register on our skin, our brain receives the information and sends a signal to move our hand away. This isn't a conscious act—we can't think this quickly. It's an instinctive response that happens in far less than a split second. Since we can't comprehend even a half second, let alone thousandths of a second, we are aware of the brain's response only after the incident.

Imagine a scenario in which there is continuous heat, only this is the kind of heat generated by people demanding something of you. In such a situation, the brain is receiving an overwhelming amount of input, all of which it seeks to act on. It begins firing at higher and higher frequencies as it tries to keep up with the demand. But we have limits to our ability to function, though we don't like to admit this. These limits are reached first on our output side because the brain can't respond as fast as information comes in. When the difference between input and output is great enough, the body starts to shake.

Drugs don't remove the imbalance. On the contrary, by masking the symptoms, they may even allow the imbalance to intensify. The person's condition, though on the surface appearing to improve, actually worsens.

A Blow to the Head

How did this woman become depressed in the first place?

Looking at her brain assessment, I asked her, "Did you experience a blow to the left rear of your head, which seems to have followed a blow to the right front? It's as if you received an upward blow while you were falling."

"That's exactly what happened," she confirmed. "I had a bicycle accident, and the first blow was to my right front. It flipped me backwards, and when I turned, it hit on the left side."

"And does this mean you are having some serious trouble with your eyes?"

"Yes," said the woman. "In fact, just last week my optometrist told me my eyes were deteriorating too fast."

"I know you are well versed in the medical field and are acquainted with people of every specialty. But what if this is all about your brain balance? We can see the imbalance. If you can balance your brain, you might be able to mitigate all these symptoms to one degree or another."

I paused for a moment, then continued, "By the way, your brain assessment indicates that about twelve to fifteen years ago, you experienced a feeling of abandonment and isolation. Is that accurate?"

The woman was stunned. "Fourteen years ago my children left

me and moved in with my ex-husband," she said. "It was devastating, and I felt completely abandoned."

"All of these things have left patterns in your brain," I explained, "but that's not a bad thing. If you hadn't been imprinted in this way, you might not have survived the incidents at the time. You have lived through them and survived, whereas many haven't. They have turned to drugs or self-destruction in some other form. Your brain did a good job—in fact, an unbelievable job. But now you need to balance it so the patterns can change to those that are more helpful in your life as it is now."

The Drawback to Antidepressants

We have become a society that relies a great deal on prescription medications. For instance, we use antidepressants to change our mood. But although we rely on them heavily, some antidepressants don't work at all.[6] Even when they do seem to help, they often lose their effectiveness over the course of treatment.[7]

Antidepressants are made to increase the chemicals known as neurotransmitters. Even when they work, it's an artificial way of changing the brain, generating activity that's not present in a normal brain. Though it may relieve the symptoms, the antidepressant doesn't cure the depression. The cause, which lies in an imbalance in the brain, is untouched by the medication.[8] In fact, the antidepressant may trigger an even greater imbalance.[9]

This is why antidepressants can lead to suicide, especially among teens and young adults.[10] Because a teen's world is so volatile, a state caused by the combination of hormones flooding the system and the psychological need to establish an identity, we never know which of the many changes they have to cope with might prove to be one too many. Hence the current advice is that certain types of antidepressants shouldn't be given to teens.

People tend to think of depression as a single syndrome, but it isn't. To say that someone has "depression" isn't a diagnosis but simply a description of how the individual feels. When the brain patterns of depressed individuals are examined, it becomes clear there isn't just one pattern associated with depression. In fact, at least sixteen dominant patterns have been detected. Were the brain of each of these individuals to be trained in the same way, the results from one to another would bear no similarity. For this reason, each brain needs a specific approach if it is to be restored to balance and harmony.

When we consider the kinds of behavior associated with depression, over a dozen different behaviors are generally labeled "depression." No antidepressant can possibly deal with all these behaviors in a single stroke, nor are they designed to do this. They are generally intended to deal with one chemical activity of the brain only, and thus often fail to address the actual cause of the individual's depression. When an antidepressant affects all areas of the brain in the same way, it can reduce the effectiveness of those areas that don't need dealing with in this way.

Brain training is much more precise, and becoming increasingly so. It looks at a person's emotional state from the vantage of the various lobes of the brain as the trainers put the brain through its paces during the assessment. Then the computer compares how the mathematical algorithms applied to this particular brain's energy patterns depict possible areas of imbalance. For instance, if one person says they are happy, while another says they are unhappy, we pay attention to the differences in the brain's energy patterns to determine which balances or imbalances may be connected to the state of happiness being experienced. We see the reasons for a person's happiness or unhappiness in the brain's activity. From observing thousands of brains, it's been possible to begin understanding how brain pattern imbalances are associated with some pathologies.

Medicated Madness

When a person abruptly cuts back on antidepressants, it may put their brain into a state of chaos. The imbalanced state of their brain is no longer being masked, and this can be a dangerous situation. It's why physicians are careful to recommend appropriate dosage reductions over time with any antidepressant.

In chapter two, we noted that Steven Kazmierczak, who opened fire on an Illinois campus, ceased taking his medication for depression two weeks before he perpetrated this atrocity. What part did this play in his crime?

In light of the advice generally given to reduce the dosage of antidepressants slowly, we might be tempted to think that when a person commits such a crime, it's because they suddenly went off their medication. But it isn't this simple.

Though people stop taking their medication for a variety of reasons, these reasons are generally rooted in the individual's discomfort. A person may be struggling to offset their imbalance, trying to do something that will improve their level of balance throughout the brain, but the medication dulls their ability to feel, which frustrates their efforts. If the person is inwardly raging, trying to break out of a parasympathetic state, they won't be able to feel the extent of their rage as long as they are medicated. Consequently, they may become even more desensitized to the world around them. They are already dissociated from their environment because their brake pedal is depressed, and the medication compounds this. On the positive side, the medication may be keeping them from harming themselves or harming anybody else. But it is simultaneously making them more uncomfortable, not less.

The same happens with stimulants and street drugs. They might alleviate a problem initially, but they hit back with a vengeance. The individual's mood undergoes a steep rise to a peak, followed by a steep drop. This leaves them feeling empty, and perhaps even frightened they are about to implode. So they take another hit in order to achieve the spike again. Only this time, because some of the drug stays in their system from the previous hit, the spike is a little higher—and the higher the spike, the worse the feeling when the drop follows. Pretty soon the person is on a merry-go-round that goes faster and faster. Their overall discomfort increases. When it reaches a critical point, they find themselves on a downward spiral that's a toboggan ride to hell.

In such a situation, a person may overdose. They may take in more of a drug than their body can handle. In some cases, they don't make it to the hospital. It's too much of a shock for their system and they die. If they do make it to the hospital, they are first detoxed, then likely sent to a substance rehabilitation program, especially in the case of use of popular street drugs. Unfortunately, drug rehabilitation programs haven't proven effective for a high percentage of addicts, which means that many of those who go through them are back for further treatment somewhere between three to twenty-four months.[11] This repeated cycle takes a toll on their body. For instance, a street drug like methamphetamine, which is a popular means of getting high, literally sucks the calcium out of the individual's teeth and bones. Crystals form beneath the skin, with sores on the skin's surface. In due course, as the person scratches their sores, crystals fall out.

Methamphetamine users are so "checked out," they don't recognize they aren't actually "in" the world in the way a person normally is. Consequently, they have little investment in their life—and with so little invested, they have no interest in going to a treatment center. The purpose of the treatment center is to free addicts from the unreality in which they are living. Since to be deprived of this unreality is the most frightening thing an addict can imagine, they usually resist treatment.

A person who abuses prescription medications doesn't want to go to a treatment center either, because as soon as they check in, they won't be able to get their prescription medications anymore. They either have to come up with a different set of excuses for why they should be given a fresh prescription, which gets harder and harder, or find a different doctor, which also becomes increasingly difficult. Little wonder such individuals often say they want to receive treatment yet actually resist entering a treatment program.

The Power of a Belief

Many of us want to solve all our problems with a pill rather than looking at the dysfunction that's causing the problems. But a problem that doesn't originate from the lack of a pill can't be solved with a pill. It can only be masked or mitigated temporarily.

People report that an antidepressant saved their life. I wouldn't argue with this for a moment. But as Dr. Bruce Lipton articulates, we have to understand how powerful a belief can be. Extensive research has shown that many claims for antidepressants simply can't be validated. In actual clinical trials with thousands of people, a sugar pill often worked as effectively as the antidepressant—and it didn't have the repercussions that antidepressants can have.[12] In such cases, the person *believed* that the pill they took could make them feel better, and their belief—not the drug or the sugar pill—brought this about.

The problem is that after a while a particular antidepressant no longer works because the body establishes immunity to it.[13] For a time, the individual feels better, but in due course the effect wears off. When the person hits the wall again, they conclude that their antidepressant is no longer working. Because they believe this, it actually doesn't work for them anymore. Since its effectiveness depends to some degree on their belief and they have concluded it doesn't work, it can't work.

When an antidepressant seems to stop working, the person is switched to a new drug. In due course the same phenomenon is likely to occur as with the first antidepressant. Drugs may help in the short term, but they are unlikely to be the solution for the long term. Hence, they are unlikely to solve the problem.

The Limitations of a Pill

There is a widespread belief that antidepressants correct brain chemistry. Is this really true?

Suppose we have a pond we wish to be a bright blue color. We can drop an appropriate quantity of blue dye into the pond until the water becomes the shade of blue we prefer. Due to exposure to the elements, especially the sun's rays, the blue may eventually fade. When it begins to do so, we can add further dye, and once again the water will be a vivid blue. In fact, the water will remain the color we wish it to be as long as we continue to add dye.

We assume antidepressants work in a similar way to adding dye to a pond. Each time we take a dose of the antidepressant, we imagine it correcting our brain chemistry much like the dye corrects the color of the pond water. Since the water remains blue as long as there is sufficient dye in the pond, we assume we will remain free of depression as long as sufficient antidepressant remains in our system.

In reality, something different happens. Unlike adding dye to a pond, no matter how much antidepressant we add, in due course it ceases to work. Were the antidepressant actually correcting brain chemistry in the way dye corrects the color of pond water, it would continue to do so. It would work each time a dose is taken.

Continually adding an antidepressant to our system doesn't work because depression isn't the result of a chemical imbalance in the brain. There *is* a chemical imbalance—you can see an imbalance in brain assessments. But the cause of the imbalance lies deeper than the mere lack of a chemical. It lies in an imbalance of the neural network, which antidepressants can't address and only mask for a while. In other words, a problem that wasn't created by the lack of a pill can't be solved with a pill.

When a person trains their brain, they address the imbalance in the network—the functional aspects of the brain—and thereby correct the cause of their difficulty. In other words, balancing the brain can affect depression at its source.

Naturally, people wonder whether we can prove this clinically, and we can. It's possible to do blood tests that reveal from biological markers how a person's chemistry has been altered. In a similar non-invasive manner, it has also been demonstrated that exercise can alleviate depression more effectively than antidepressants. When exercise and antidepressants were compared over the course of a few weeks, both proved to be about equally helpful in alleviating depression. But as the trial progressed into months, exercise was shown to be the more helpful. [14]

People whose brain becomes balanced not only feel excited about life, they tend to sleep more soundly and have more energy. For instance, a woman had been sleeping nine or ten hours a night and still felt tired in the morning. When she began training her brain, she found she slept only five or six hours, yet she awakened rested and felt great all day. "What's wrong with me?" she wondered when she simply couldn't sleep longer. Of course, this woman had been sleeping nine or ten hours because she had been depressed for years. Now that she wasn't depressed, she didn't require as much sleep. If someone is going to bed and falling asleep in reasonable time—without passing out from the effects of alcohol or exhaustion—and awakening rested after only five, six, or seven hours, this is good news.

I hypothesize that brain function drives brain chemistry. Previous medical science would contend that the chemistry drives the function. Someday, should the walls come down so that the new technology is utilized alongside the old science, we will probably find that a combination of the two approaches enables a knockout blow for afflictions such as anxiety and depression. I envision that an optimized future treatment will likely involve the use of a combination of pharmaceuticals and brain training—much like depression today is often treated with antidepressants and cognitive therapy. Initially, pharmaceuticals would be used to stabilize the person until the full effects of brain training are felt. From this point on, the individual would be monitored so that the quantity of the pharmaceuticals can be reduced, perhaps even allowing the individual to be weaned off medication altogether.

The problem with long-term dependence on drugs is that, while appearing to solve one problem, they often create another. For instance, after the drug Wellbutrin was developed to alleviate addiction to nicotine, subsequent studies of its effect revealed that nicotine users who were also depressed found their depression improved. So Wellburin began to be prescribed for depression.

Later, it was discovered that it has a number of negative side affects—cardiac arrhythmias, dizziness, constipation, nausea, dry mouth, blurred vision, and so on.[15] For this reason, follow-ups with a physician are deemed appropriate.[16]

If pharmaceuticals are used primarily as a bridge until brain training has a chance to address the root of the problem, the client receives maximum benefit in the short term, together with a minimum of side effects over the longer haul.

When the science of the future addresses an individual's body, mind, and spirit, and not just a single aspect of our humanity, it will lead to optimizing the whole of our being. Physically, psychologically, and spiritually, our lives will exude balance and harmony. How soon this will happen on a wide scale is unclear, but it's where the flow of our information and technology is leading us.

14

Can You Trust Yourself?

TRUST IS BEDROCK TO HUMAN CIVILIZATION, and indeed to all of our interaction as a species. If we didn't trust, we would never set foot outside our home. We would never flip an electrical switch, never eat anything we didn't grow ourselves, never set foot in a car, and certainly never board an aircraft.

To trust is natural for a human with a balanced brain. If a pregnancy and birth have gone well, when we are infants we exhibit a high level of trust. Of course, it's vital we trust because, as infants, we can do nothing whatever for ourselves and must assume others will take care of everything needful for our survival.

In the natural course of things, this innocent trust would continue unabated throughout childhood, the teen years, and into adulthood. Sadly, in few of us does life unfold in a manner that has a perfect and unobstructed flow. Instead, our lives are punctuated by the disruption caused by trauma, environmental factors, and genetically inherited vulnerabilities. This disruption tends to unbalance the brain and hence disrupt our natural proclivity to trust.

As trust evaporates, depression rushes in to fill the void.

A Personal Y2K

When events happened in her personal life that she couldn't make sense of, a medical doctor found herself experiencing increasing difficulty functioning in everyday life. Something traumatic seemed to happen to this doctor about every three weeks.

"Everyone was worried about what was going to happen with the approach of Y2K," she recalls. "Well, starting January 1, 2000, I experienced my own Y2K. I had been working as a medical doctor and was laid off from the clinic of which I was a part. It was particularly distressing because my husband at the time didn't have an income either."

Shortly thereafter her stepmother passed away. Her father, who was 87, clearly couldn't cope with the loss of his wife. Occurring as it did at this juncture in her career, this was to become a huge challenge for Dr. Karyn.

When Dr. Karyn opened her own clinic, she developed a breast discharge that had an abnormal color. While she was pondering what this meant, her husband announced, "There is somebody else, and I want to marry her."

As far as Dr. Karyn could tell, she and her husband got along much better than most couples ever get along. Already reeling from everything that had been happening in her life, this announcement came as an immense shock. "My husband was sitting in a chair several feet from me," she relates, "and I could see his lips moving, but it was as if his voice came from behind me." Unable to bear what was happening, she was dissociating from the reality she was facing. With no fight left in her and nowhere to flee for security, she simply went into a freeze response.

That night she began sobbing and couldn't stop. As she plowed through a full schedule of patients the following day, she found herself sobbing between appointments. In the past, patients had described to her a condition in which, following a trauma such as a divorce, they simply couldn't eat. Now she experienced this herself. She was completely without appetite, and everything she tried to force down tasted like cardboard and went down with the texture of sandpaper. All she could consume was soup.

Dr. Karyn had believed her husband was crazy about her. She always felt she was on a pedestal. They hardly ever argued. She believed they had a close relationship. That this man she had trusted most wanted to leave her for another woman—his "soul mate," as he put it—seemed to her bizarre. How could he feel this way when he acted as though she walked on water? "The whole experience felt surreal," she mused.

As the inevitability of the end of their marriage sank in, it felt to Dr. Karyn as if everything in the world around her that normally was bright and beautiful had taken on a grey tone. Nothing excited her. Nothing even interested her anymore, not even the work that was her life and soul.

A deep depression settled in. Realizing she couldn't see patients any longer because she was finding it impossible to make sound decisions, Dr. Karyn closed her medical practice. "I couldn't even think my way out of a paper bag," she recalls, "let alone think clearly enough to help patients." The emotional trauma had triggered a protective brain pattern in which she could no longer trust her judgment. "I was way beyond doubting myself," she explains.

"Everything I thought was real now seemed as if it might not be real at all. It was as if my whole world had been flipped over."

The essential trust that makes human life viable had been shattered for Dr. Karyn. On top of this, she discovered she had a cancerous tumor that required a mastectomy.

It had been a year from hell.

A Turnaround

Life was difficult following a mastectomy in early 2001. A good day for Dr. Karyn was when she managed to get out of bed, shower, dress, and eat. After some months, she began working in a medical practice with a colleague three days a week. Between patients and over lunch, a year after her world blew apart, she was still sobbing.

A pharmacist suggested the doctor check her thyroid. It was in the mid range, only slightly low. Nevertheless, she began taking thyroid medication. Almost immediately she felt as though she was climbing out of a black hole.

She was now seeing two therapists a week, but the counseling was only minimally helpful. She tried various other therapies. The thyroid medication was the only thing that made any real difference.

In their divorce, Dr. Karyn had lost her dance partner, her business partner, her husband, and her best friend in a single stroke. One of the doctor's therapists suggested she start seeking out things she could delight in—a bird, a butterfly, or some kind of activity that would brighten her mood. At this time, when the world seemed completely grey, it was difficult for Dr. Karyn to find anything in her surroundings that elevated her spirit.

In her own practice again at last, the doctor appeared to most people to be functioning quite normally. Out of public view, she still felt a great loss of confidence and a continuous ache in her chest. Not only her chest, but also her arms felt heavy, and she even had difficulty standing up straight and holding her head up. As she walked, she gave the appearance of someone who had caved in from her sadness. Bathed in trauma for what felt like an eternity now, her body had felt too uncomfortable for her to be in it. Consequently, she dissociated from much of the bodily sensation she was experiencing. It was as if she was experiencing an almost continual out-of-body state.

Many of us learn to live with the sadness that enters our life. We develop a modicum of happiness and we get by. For Dr. Karyn, several years would pass during which, although she seemed to function, she was unable to find the joy in life for which she longed.

Replanting Trust

In September 2007, Dr. Karyn was introduced to brain training by a friend. Her brain assessment before training showed that her parasympathetic nervous system was functioning at twice the level of her sympathetic nervous system. It was clear from this assessment that the heartache she had felt for seven years was a result of the constraint placed on her by this heavy parasympathetic dominance. It was as if her physical functioning had a brake pedal engaged, which she experienced as a heavy load.

This explains why, following brain training, a friend described her as "a party girl without alcohol." In no time at all, her friends all recognized she was a different person—laughing, smiling, able to focus, and able to make direct contact with people in a way she hadn't in a long time. She was also sleeping more soundly.

The most important change was that the doctor was once again feeling a sense of hope, and her spirit was more buoyant. In fact, in the wake of training her brain, the ache in her chest had diminished by about ninety percent.

The upbeat spirit that began to pervade Dr. Karyn's life spilled over into her medical office. She was once again able to devote herself to the work she loves, and her several staff members enjoy the light and fun atmosphere of the clinic.

With patients, Dr. Karyn finds herself more present. She listens to every detail in a way she didn't before, which has enabled her to become increasingly accurate in her diagnoses. As long as she was depressed, it wasn't only her mood that suffered but her ability to think clearly and quickly. Her new lucidity means she finds herself able to explain to patients more clearly what's happening to them.

At some time in the past, Dr. Karyn had suffered a minor stroke that affected her coordination. Going down her office steps, she had to hold onto the handrail and walk carefully. Whenever she was on the dance floor, she found she couldn't spin with the coordination she once enjoyed. She also found she couldn't balance in heels—in fact, she had given up wearing heels years ago. Yet, after brain training, she could run down the stairs at her office in three-inch heels without holding onto the handrail! In other words, her brain's new balance and harmony was also reflected in her physical coordination.

Though Dr. Karyn at times still feels mild anxiety, and continues to train her brain periodically, the panic attacks that caused her to gasp for breath all ceased. As a close friend tells her, "You have so much going for you now."

Her friend explained that she also laughs from a different place. Before, her dominant emotion was depression, so her friends tried to get her to laugh. When she laughed, it was in a restricted manner and accompanied by heaviness—laughter tinged with sadness. As a result of training her brain, she has less muscular-skeletal spasm, and hence not only laughs more freely but stands more erect with her head held higher. Even her walk exhibits greater confidence.

The Centrality of Trust

Trust is fundamental to our enjoyment of life. A violation of trust can leave us feeling incapable of enjoying life and even rob us of the will to live.

Though trust is a given for a balanced brain when it starts out on life's voyage, our journey through childhood is often precarious where trust is concerned. Those we look to for reinforcement of our sense of who we are—our external mirrors—often let us down. The very ones we anticipate receiving love from raise their voices in anger, and sometimes even strike us physically, causing us bodily pain and mental anguish. We learn that the world isn't as safe as we might wish, and our ability to trust becomes tempered with caution, if not outright fear.

If, despite the disappointments of growing up, we manage to retain sufficient faith in humanity to entrust ourselves, starry-eyed, to another person in a committed relationship, we anticipate that it will be "forever." But like Dr. Karyn, almost half of us live to experience the shattering of our trust through divorce, as love seems to die on the vine, while many who manage to stay together do so in a fashion that's less than joyous. Thus, in one way or another, somewhere along the way we all experience a rude awakening to how untrustworthy our trust in others can be.

While a balanced brain is a trusting brain, this trust has to mature until it's centered neither in another person nor in a particular set of circumstances, but solely in our own essence—in a brain in which our consciousness and our brain patterns are aligned to create self-trust.

When people are vulnerable, they lead with their wounds, and they are drawn to people with the same wounds. In the long term, two individuals with the same wounds and vulnerability don't benefit each other. Unless they deal with their pain, they etch the pathways of the pain deeper. When people are balanced, they become resilient and can open up because they aren't afraid of being lampooned if the other person doesn't like what they reveal. Balanced individuals are not dependent on others for a joyful life.

When Life Falls Apart

There are many people for whom life falls apart, just as it did in the case of Dr. Karyn. When such individuals train their brain, again and again they discover a new level of competence that gives them the trust, confidence, and courage to put their life back together.

I want to conclude this chapter by sharing with you just one other woman's experience when her dreams were shattered by divorce followed by the loss of her career. She wrote to me:

> When I first heard about brain conditioning, I was in a crisis personally, emotionally, and financially. I had been separated from my husband for a little over a month and I felt like my life was falling apart. I felt overwhelmed, depressed, and full of fear about my future. I cried off and on all day long, barely functioning.
>
> Besides separating from my husband, I was worried about losing my job because the mortgage industry I worked in was

collapsing. My income had already dropped to about a third of what it was usually, and companies were closing daily. Later in January, I was laid off with no prospect of getting another job in my industry.

I started doing brain conditioning sessions because I was trying everything that I could find to stabilize myself, not because I knew or understood the technology or what was supposed to happen. I just knew I needed help, and I was determined to do whatever I could to find relief. My goals had to do with managing my anxiety, wanting a sense of happiness and well-being, and to improve sleep.

I did not really know what to expect and I didn't really feel like anything was different during the time that I did the sessions, doing ten at first, skipping about two weeks, then coming back for four more sessions.

Somewhere around two weeks after the training, I woke up one morning and my mind was quiet. At that point I realized that all the negative mind chatter and racing thoughts were no longer there. For as far back as I can remember, my mind was actually quiet for the first time. What an incredible blessing this was.

I had always said that my mind was my friend, but it was more often my enemy. It served me well when I needed it intellectually or for problem solving, but it also tortured me with obsessive thoughts that I could not get out of my head. I could redirect the thoughts for a few minutes, but then they would come right back.

I also started to sleep for longer periods. I usually can fall asleep okay, but I used to wake up often, especially when I was stressed out. Now, I would only wake up once or twice instead of every hour on the hour, and I could go right back to sleep.

Next I started to notice there were longer and longer periods of time during which I experienced relief from my anxiety, and I began to feel peaceful and calm most of the time.

It's been almost six months since I first did brain conditioning. I just realized another huge change that has come from the training. For most of my life I didn't like to read books. I have been an audio learner instead of reading because it was easier for me to assimilate what I was hearing. In the past month I have read four books, one of which was particularly challenging because it was about cell biology and I had never taken many sciences when I was in school. For the first time, I was able to read books because my mind was quiet and I could focus and concentrate on what I was reading. This makes me very happy and I continue to read about a book a week.

Every one of the issues that I had in the past has been improved since having brain training sessions. The quality of my life has improved and I have been able to handle my difficult situations calmly and without panic and fear.

15

Beyond Post-Traumatic Stress

ONE OF THE MOST RESISTANT OF HUMAN CONDITIONS is post-traumatic stress disorder. When an individual is stricken with this pathology, it's like plunging into a bottomless abyss. As Vietnam War veteran Mick Patrick DeBriwere put it, "PTSD is like a wormhole between two worlds. I am not sure there are any remedial interventions that will permanently solve that dark night of the soul."

Mick had pretty much given up hope of ever being free of post-traumatic stress disorder when he learned of brain training. He underwent years of suffering before he was finally diagnosed in 1997 with "chronic post-traumatic stress disorder, coupled with the complications of multiple head injuries and medical problems related to exposure to Agent Orange."

Mick's diagnosis came after what he describes as "twenty-eight years of psychic numbing." During those years, he explored an array of treatments, not only as a patient but also as a certified Gestalt therapist. His journey in search of healing took him into Transactional Analysis, Rolfing, EST, Co-counseling, EMDR, Hypnosis, Transcendental Meditation, and on countless spiritual retreats. None of these approaches brought real healing. "I can assure you the symptoms of post-traumatic stress disorder flow like a river beneath all of these structured approaches to a healthy mind," Mick says. "The residual aspects of PTSD seem to have subterranean aspects that don't lend themselves to conventional remedies."

In his years in the United States Marine Corps, Mick was with the 7th Marines in Quang Nam Province of the Republic of Vietnam, an area known for its heavy casualties. Since his return from Vietnam in 1969, he has become a member of the Marine Corps League, American Legion, and Veterans of Foreign Wars. Currently, he spends much of his time mentoring young combat veterans and conducting workshops for post-traumatic stress disorder.

"As a person who has meditated for thirty-six years," Mick recounts, "I have always derived the benefits of Transcendental Meditation: lower blood pressure, more focus, and a state of tranquility. All very subjective. Interestingly, the protocols of brain training are able to capture that subjective mind state, objectify and quantify it by allowing me to witness the exact nature of the accompanying frequency of brain waves, while simultaneously experiencing that state of being. And then, in turn, learning how to enhance that very state. Now this is training at a level simply not accessible by way of conventional therapy!"

Mick's experience of the limited ability of a variety of modalities to heal post-traumatic stress disorder mirrors my own. As I have already indicated, following a traumatic event, I too found myself suffering from post-traumatic stress disorder, and it was finally only through the discovery of brain training that I was able to become free of this condition. My personal experience echoes that of Mick, who concluded, "I would recommend this vanguard technology to anyone, without reservation, particularly my battle buddies. I hope to return for an encore."

He added, "I say, 'Bottle it!'"

The Birth of Brain Training

A fight-or-flight response that continues over a long period has serious repercussions. It can lead to such symptoms as hypertension, rapid arrhythmia, panic attacks, outbursts of anger, chronic anxiety, irritation, depression, high cholesterol, heart disease, stroke, type one diabetes, digestive problems, sleep problems, cold hands and cold feet, difficulty concentrating, and blurring of vision when focusing on something, such as reading.

In other words, while post-traumatic stress results in an increase in heart rate, blood pressure, fuel availability, adrenalin release, oxygen circulation to vital organs, blood clotting, and pupil size, it also produces a decrease in sexual response, together with a reduced capacity for fuel storage and insulation activity. Because post-traumatic stress disorder can result in so much physical and mental damage, it's essential that sufferers find relief.

As somebody who has experienced post-traumatic stress disorder, I found myself experiencing outbursts of anger. It took little to anger me, and my anger, once kindled, was quick to be expressed. Again and again I told myself, "Reacting this way isn't helpful. It's costing you relationships and friendships. Nobody wants to be around you. Why can't you just stop erupting at every little provocation?" But do you think I could change my tendency to react? No, I couldn't change it. I was imprisoned by it.

Another way people respond when they find themselves behaving in ways they can't control is to turn to an outside source for the power they believe they lack. A person may seek help from what many call their Higher Power. They may pray, "God, I don't like the way I react. I know it's not helpful. Will you take this anger from me?" Millions upon millions pray such prayers. I prayed such prayers for years. Yet, like so many, I remained angry, venting my anger again and again, from year to year.

Millions who have tried to free themselves from post-traumatic stress disorder can testify that, by using standard approaches, there's seldom a way to "get out of jail free."

The answer isn't outside of us, but within us. For within is where we interface with universal consciousness. It's the natural tranquility of the brain when it's connected to its source in universal consciousness that alone can free us, and it's this that brain training can enable us to tap into.

How Post-Traumatic Stress Becomes a Disorder

It isn't possible for any of us to go through life without experiencing a measure of trauma. Whether in the form of the death of a loved one, a physical injury, being in or witnessing a car accident, or experiencing the pain of the termination of a relationship, we all endure a measure of trauma.

Suppose you are in a car accident in which you survive but you lose a loved one. Because the pain is excruciating, you can barely function. Recognizing this, for a time society allows you to grieve. But generally it's not very long before people start telling you, "Get over it." What society doesn't realize is that in many such cases the brain has been seriously altered by shock.

How do you "get over" a trauma if your brain has been drastically changed by the experience? How do you simply "move on" if your father or mother, brother or sister dies in your arms after an accident?

Or take the case of a teen, newly qualified to drive, passing through an intersection when a truck is barreling down a hill and doesn't see the stop sign. Catching sight of the truck at the last minute, the teen freezes instead of stepping on the brake and is almost killed in the pile up. How does the teen "get over" this? Although medical help arrives quickly and people comfort the victim, none of this addresses the individual's inner state.

Even if we never experience a tragedy of this kind personally, all of us are exposed to trauma in the wake of terrorist attacks on various nations, together with natural disasters such as an earthquake, a tsunami, or a hurricane, as these events are played and replayed endlessly on television news. For instance, how many times have we seen the Twin Towers collapse, even if we were nowhere near the scene? The stress of a single incident can be deeply traumatizing when we replay it over and over.

Because we've all lived through traumatic events, almost every human carries within them a measure of post-traumatic stress. But it doesn't reach the level of a "disorder" in most of us because the trauma isn't generally piled one traumatic experience upon another in the compressed time frame that happens in a disaster or war zone.

In war, people are exposed in a short space of time to more traumatic experiences than most of us normally experience in a lifetime. Under such circumstances, the brain generates a dominant pattern of fight-or-flight. The Associated Press reported, "Roughly one in every five U.S. troops who have survived the bombs and other dangers of Iraq and Afghanistan now suffers from major depression or post-traumatic stress, an independent study said Thursday. It estimated the toll at 300,000 or more."[17]

A particularly striking example is a member of the armed forces who returned from Iraq suffering from post-traumatic stress. During his tour of duty, this soldier spent much of his time on mobile patrol, watching for vehicles that might contain a bomb. Lone cars parked along the roadside were especially suspicious. Time and again he witnessed those cars exploding, and more than once the explosion ended the life of a friend. So now, back home, whenever he sees a lone car parked on the side of the road—especially if it's an older car—he's likely to react in an unpredictable manner. Sometimes he takes extreme action, such as swerving across several lanes of traffic to get away from the parked vehicle because his neural network tells him it might blow up at any moment.

If we remind a soldier who has returned from duty that he is back in his home country, we are giving him information he already knows all too well. Logically, he knows that to veer across several lanes of traffic makes no sense. Having grown up in North America, he has known all his life that a car sitting on the side of the road isn't likely to blow up. Still, he endangers himself, his family, and other drivers because his logic isn't running the show. His traumatized, unbalanced brain is in charge, and he reacts based on its imbalance.

Was the reactionary pattern of the veteran helpful to him in Iraq? Indeed it was. But now, back home, it's a danger to him—to the point that he could end up causing a fatal traffic accident. This is because the soldier returned to society in a state of hypersensitivity. Because super-vigilance saved the soldier's life at one time, it becomes a dominant brain pattern that plays out every moment of every day. Many returning soldiers find themselves wary of everything, forever on the lookout for some kind of threat. Their sympathetic nervous system is in overdrive, with the consequence that they cannot relax. This is one of the symptoms exhibited by soldiers returning from battle who experience post-traumatic stress disorder.

The hyper-vigilance experienced by service personnel and others returning from Iraq and Afghanistan is particularly acute—more so than was the case with soldiers returning from Vietnam. In the Vietnam War, soldiers went out on a foray, looking for the enemy. In Iraq and Afghanistan, they are among the enemy all the time, and consequently 24/7 under the gun. They never know whether the person next to them in a market may blow them up. Even an innocent-looking child who walks up to them may be harboring explosives. Is it any wonder soldiers experience severe post-traumatic stress disorder in huge numbers? The problem is compounded by the fact that if service personnel tell their superiors they are experiencing emotional problems, they may be accused of cowardice and ostracized by their peers. If they refuse to go on patrol, they may be arrested.

The Straw that Breaks the Camel's Back

Despite the severity of post-traumatic stress disorder on the modern battlefield, it isn't unrelated to the trauma daily life puts us through. We can see this from the case of an Air Force fighter pilot who served from 1991 to 2003, including twenty-seven combat missions over Iraq. Years after he left the service, he discovered that he suffered from post-traumatic stress disorder. Instead of sleeping soundly, he awakened multiple times during the night, which meant he rarely felt rested in the morning. His inability to sleep well was accompanied by hyper-vigilance and a short fuse. At the outset of brain training, the former pilot scored twenty-two on both the Beck Depression Inventory and the Beck Anxiety Inventory—scores that are moderately high.

However, war wasn't this pilot's first brush with trauma. The son of emotionally abusive alcoholic parents, he grew up tense and tried to control his environment by eliminating any and all mistakes, a form of perfectionism. He also sought to protect himself emotionally by remaining aloof and avoiding intimate relationships. His experience in a war zone simply magnified the tension and distrust that was already ingrained in him.

A soldier's formative experiences may lay the groundwork for post-traumatic stress disorder. The degree to which a soldier has been subjected to trauma while growing up often adds to the possibility that the stress the individual carries in themselves before they ever go to war will develop into a disorder on the battlefield.

Another military man, who joined the Marine Corps at age seventeen, was injured during a tour in Vietnam as a machine gun squad leader. While in medical care in Okinawa, his appendix ruptured. When he finally recovered, he was discharged and declared disabled with post-traumatic stress disorder.

As was the case with the pilot mentioned earlier, the post-traumatic stress disorder suffered by this marine had its roots in his earlier life. When he was two days old, he was put up for adoption by his mother. He later learned she tried to abort the pregnancy by drinking turpentine and hitting herself in the abdomen. His adoptive parents were good people, but it was his adoptive sister who provided his most meaningful support. However, when he was five years old, the sister left the household to marry—a traumatic event that caused him to feel abandoned. On top of this, his adoptive parents divorced when he was eleven. The long-established brain imbalance resulting from these issues was a perfect setup for the onset of post-traumatic stress disorder in the wake of the shock of injury in Vietnam.

In the case of both the pilot and the marine, a measure of relief came almost immediately when they each started to train their brain. For instance, the inability to sleep had been a serious problem for the marine. In addition to waking several times during the night, he was plagued by night terrors. When he began training his brain, he reported, "I slept an entire eight hours last night straight through. That is the first time I can remember sleeping through the night since I was a kid."

The pilot also experienced relief. After training his brain over the course of a single week, he scored a one on the Beck Depression Inventory and eleven, considered mild, on the Anxiety Inventory. He reported feeling calm and relaxed for the first time in years. "Of all the things I've tried since leaving the military," he concluded, "this has been the most significant. Thank you for this tremendous gift."

Post-Traumatic Stress Disorder Needn't Be a Life Sentence

How post-traumatic stress disorder generally results from a buildup of stressful events rather than from a single traumatic incident is graphically illustrated in the case of Skip Flynn, a Roman Catholic priest with a doctorate in clinical psychology.

In 1973, Skip became a political prisoner in Chile's famous *Estadio Nacional*—National Football (soccer) Stadium—when he was sentenced to the firing squad. Fortunately, his religious order, family, friends, and political connections put pressure on the United States government to negotiate his release. When he returned to his home in Florida, he earned his doctorate and became a Certified Addiction specialist, a role he fulfills to this day. Although he was effective in the work he was doing, his own life exhibited symptoms that dated back to his brush with death in

Chile. For instance, he found himself unable to fly without Valium. He also manifested a non-Parkinson's involuntary tremor.

In his capacity as an addiction specialist, Skip was always on the lookout for effective tools to help his clients. In due course, friends who had heard about brain training mentioned it to him and he decided to explore it.

Skip's initial assessment revealed that although the Chile incident deeply affected him, this alone wasn't the reason for his present symptoms. Rather, it was the accumulation over the years of one stressful episode after another, augmented by the trauma of the firing squad, that precipitated the onset of post-traumatic stress disorder.

It's often the case that a person's tension grows and grows until even a single episode, sometimes even something quite small, becomes the proverbial straw that breaks the camel's back.

Although Skip had managed his initial trauma without coming apart at the seams, it had all finally become too much for him. His brain was putting so much energy into holding its stressful pattern at bay that it simply had no spare energy to cope with yet another stressful incident. Think of it in terms of tilting a table with an object on it. If the table is tilted far enough, the object loses its grip and slides off. Similarly, when the brain reaches a certain point of imbalance, it too loses its grip and the result is post-traumatic stress disorder .

In his very first brain training session, Skip saw his tremor vanish. After a week of training, he also flew back to Florida with no Valium at all and has flown Valium-free ever since. How could so little brain training accomplish so much?

Imagine a conversation between yourself and another person, in which the other party has no knowledge of the facts of a particular situation but you aren't free to divulge what you know. As the conversation progresses, you realize the other party is completely mistaken in their conclusions. Because their opinion is so offensive, you find yourself becoming angry. But, forbidden to reveal the truth, you have to hold it in. As the conversation progresses, it requires more and more energy to keep from exclaiming, "You have no idea what you're talking about!" In fact, maintaining the imbalance may generate such high energy that you find yourself trembling. The situation is akin to a plane with propellers revved up at high speed while the aircraft's brakes are on. The plane literally shakes from the energy being held back.

Skip's case was similar to this. When he began training his brain, the energy imbalance he had been experiencing dropped dramatically so that his tremor and fear of flying went away. Skip also had a severe case of tinnitus, a ringing in his ears that resulted from several car accidents over the years. After training his brain, he estimated the ringing to be diminished by seventy-five percent.

Skip's business partner commented on how he walks differently and carries himself differently today. The tension in his body has gone, so that he actually looks more relaxed. Gone too are the aches and pains he experienced each morning upon arising. As a consequence, Skip and his partner have incorporated brain training into their work.

16

Are You Ready to Embrace
Your Real Identity?

WE HAVE A TENDENCY TO RELATE to other people most easily based on what we have in common with them. Sometimes, what we have in common with someone is our wounds. To relate based on wounds for a short while can be helpful if it carries us through the period when we are severely affected by these wounds. It acts as a boat to take us across the river of our initial pain. But woe be to us if we don't disembark when we reach the other side.

Many times people don't get off at the other side of the river after their initial shock and anguish. They hold onto their wounds until these wounds become part of their identity. There isn't a day when the wounds don't invade their experience in some form or other.

As long as a person dwells on their wounds, they affirm and fortify the brainwave pattern the brain established to get them through the crisis that caused the wound. This pattern becomes so deeply etched into the brain that the person never really gets out of crisis. They live their life with an imbalance, and they pay a huge price in terms of their happiness and their health.

The good news is that if a wounded person's brainwaves become balanced, their identity as a victim usually fades and is replaced by a sense of limitless potential.

Beyond a Victim Mentality

As a parent of two children—a son who works just down the hallway from my office and a daughter in Chicago—I cannot begin to comprehend what parents experience when they lose a child. It's an event that's unbelievably tragic.

In an attempt to deal with such a tragedy, bereaved parents often join a support group, which can initially be helpful. The emotions people go through at such a time can be so overwhelming that they experience a unique form of isolation, almost as if they were cut off from normal life. The death of a child is not a normal thing. The family and friends of most bereaved parents haven't experienced this kind of loss in their own lives and hence can't know what it means to have lost a child. By connecting with people who have been through this experience, bereaved parents realize they are not alone in their grief after all. To be around others who have survived the desperation and hopelessness they are experiencing is a great solace.

While attending a support group for some months can help a parent through the initial grief and recovery, it's common to find people still attending the support group many years after their loss. And how do they introduce themselves to the group week after week, year after year? "Hi. I'm a surviving parent, and my child was killed in an automobile accident." Their tragedy becomes their identity. Instead of seeing the tragedy as part of their life, it becomes the centerpiece of their life. They are chained to it. Indeed, the tragedy is perpetuated and magnified, so that it affects every-body in their world. They are *known* by this event. They are "the Simpsons, who lost their daughter." In other words, instead of using the group as a school from which they can graduate, they repeat the class from year to year.

When people go through a trauma of such severity, they need to be able to find an identity in the present moment, away from the experience of the past. This is what brain training can accom-plish. When the brain is balanced, traumatized individuals start to see themselves for who they are instead of in the shadow of their tragedy. They realize, "Those things happened to me, but they aren't who I am." They again live in the present, which is life-transforming.

An Identity Based on Trauma

In the early 1990s, I had become stuck in a brain pattern that wasn't truly who I was at all. I have already described how this dele-terious pattern imprisoned me in a mindset that for ten long years robbed me of the fullness of life.

The event that triggered this brain pattern took place in San Francisco, where I helped start a program called the Friendship Banquet. Supported by the congregation of St. Paulus Lutheran Church, we served meals, without charge, to people suffering from HIV. Guests were treated in the manner of an upscale restaurant. We dressed well, ushered them to their tables, which were laid with a tablecloth, flowers, silver, and china, and served them a three-to-five-course meal. The Jewish Women's League and many of the Bay Area churches supported the program.

It was around four o'clock one afternoon and we had just finished cleaning up from the banquet. An alley led from Gough Street to the back of the church, where some boys, ages fourteen or fifteen, were milling about. I asked them if they would mind going out onto the street as I had to lock the gate. I didn't notice that one had a baseball bat.

As I was locking the gate, I felt a whoosh of air from the bat just before it hit me and knocked me to the ground. I struggled back to my feet, but then caught the next swing on my left shoulder and fell to the ground again. Even though the other three boys were kicking me, somehow I got back on my feet.

When the bat hit me yet again, one of the boys yelled, "He's down. Kill him!" I knew I had to get up again or I was going to stay down for a very long time. But no sooner was I on my feet than the bat hit me on my right cheek just under my eye. The force was so great, the bat flew out of the boy's hand, and as I fell, I landed on top of it. I grabbed it, and as I pushed myself up with it, my assailants took off.

On the x-ray table at Mount Zion Hospital that night, I was in so much pain, I just gave up and everything went dark. It wasn't an unpleasant feeling. In fact, I felt wonderful, just as many have described in a near-death experience. I wanted to leave this life but wasn't allowed to, which angered me!

By the time I came around, my head had swollen up like a balloon. I was given a morphine pump, which I appreciated. The x-rays revealed I needed surgery, so the following day I was moved to the University of California San Francisco Hospital. On the journey, a ray of sunshine burst through the clouds, symbolic of my feeling a hundred times better by the time I arrived. In the hours that followed, I learned that I wasn't going to require surgery after all.

I had always thought of myself as a kind and generous person. It's why I liked to be of service to people who were suffering, such as those who are HIV positive. But after experiencing this trauma, I found myself behaving in a manner that was completely out of line with the kind of person I had always wanted to be. To say the least, I was enraged.

When the hospital discharged me, I took a cab back to the street where the assault occurred. I knelt down. My blood was still on the sidewalk. I spat on it, then used my finger to paint my face as if I was going on a warpath. For several weeks I went looking for those young guys almost every night. Thank God we didn't encounter each other!

Over the next ten years, I played the role of the wounded one. I told myself over and over, "All I was trying to do was be a good guy. To be assaulted while doing something good is so unfair!"

As a result of the assault, one of my shoulders was partially frozen during those ten years. Why did it take a decade for it to heal? It didn't heal because I didn't really *want* it to heal. You see, it had become part of my identity. I lit up whenever somebody asked me, "What's wrong with your shoulder?" because it gave me a reason to tell my story. The story made me feel like I was a survivor of an unfair occurrence.

One therapy involved going back and working through everything associated with the assault, with the goal in mind that I would eventually be able to let go of the feelings that surrounded it by repositioning my feelings about it. Some modalities involved asking me to replay the event in my head while using certain eye movements that were intended to break the pattern of association. Some asked me to think through the situation using logic to separate my thoughts from the feelings associated with the event. Some required me to reflect on my life and feelings in general, while still others asked me to engage in such reflection with the help of medication to lessen my anxiety or alleviate my depression. But ten years later, I was *still* talking and talking about my feelings, still suffering from post-traumatic stress. Was I destined to spend a lifetime struggling to get beyond the effects of the assault?

Rehearsing Our Story

I didn't know it in those days, but there is ample evidence that not only is the repeated retelling of a traumatic event totally unnecessary, it can actually be more harmful than helpful. Repeatedly retelling what happened, and evoking the emotions and thoughts associated with it, can etch the memory of the trauma deeper and make it even more difficult to let go.

When I started training my brain, and also began working with a personal athletic trainer at the gym, my shoulder became unfrozen. Whereas before I couldn't move my shoulder—couldn't even get out onto the dance floor and dance well—I was again able to raise both my arms in a normal manner.

As a result of training my brain, I came to see the attack all those years ago in a different light. The simple fact is that people usually only carry out such hostile acts when they have a severe brain imbalance. Once we realize this, we become very understanding of and compassionate toward people who do terrible things. We realize it's the imbalance that's causing their behavior, and not who they really are. The real tragedy wasn't that I was assaulted, but that three young men had such an imbalance in their brain that they could carry out such an assault. It wasn't my tragedy, it was theirs, because they were experiencing a state of mind they had to live with unrelentingly—a state that was making them miserable and hence mad at the world.

A trauma doesn't have to become our identity, and it doesn't have to rob us of our life. In fact, after training my brain, for a little while I felt really, really sad. This sadness came from the realization I had spent an entire decade of my life looking backwards. Three minutes of my life had been allowed to dictate my future.

I also realized that there was a purpose for the suffering I went through. It led to the development of a technology that is changing the lives of people all over the planet, which makes everything I experienced worthwhile.

17

Brain Training Puts You
in Charge of Your Life

IN ALL KINDS OF AREAS OF LIFE, training our brain restores to us the ability to take responsibility for our life instead of being driven by impulses we can't control.

For instance, a woman reported, "I simply must have a half-pound of chocolate-coated almonds during my lunch hour. It's something I do every day."

"You have to have a half-pound of chocolate-coated almonds every lunch hour?" I asked, taken aback.

"Yes. If I don't, I totally self-destruct by mid afternoon. And by 5 PM, I'm ready to kill someone!"

Feeling a compulsion to eat a half-pound of chocolate-coated almonds a day may seem trivial, but any kind of compulsion can wreak havoc with our life, even when it appears inconsequential to others.

I asked this woman to set aside a certain period of time during which she wouldn't eat almonds. "Can you go for a day?" I suggested. "Just one day."

On the day the client agreed to skip the almonds, we began training. At the end of a week of training, this woman was making a half-pound of almonds last a whole week.

With a balanced brain, we are driving the bus—the bus isn't driving us. This imparts a sense of personal power. By regaining control of our life, we are able to make different choices and enjoy the freedom of living a life in balance and harmony. Whether we are eating or drinking, brain training enables us to engage in these pleasures without being obsessed.

Take Charge of Your Alcohol Consumption

The high level of alcoholism among humans is witness to how many people live their life in a state of serious brain imbalance.

There is an urgent need for effective solutions to alcoholism because of its devastating impact on society. The effects of alcoholism on health are far-reaching, affecting every system in the body and resulting in a wide range of health problems. Alcoholism can lead to memory problems, difficulty with balance, hypertension, heart disease, arrhythmia, cancer, blood disorders, hepatitis, cirrhosis of the liver, a lowered immunity to infection, gastrointestinal problems, lowered fertility, and weak bones.

On a personal level, alcoholism results in relationship troubles, child and spousal abuse, depression, and a variety of social ills such as unemployment, homelessness, suicide, self-injury, and violence including murder. Alcohol is also a factor in half of all deaths from motor vehicle accidents. In fact, about 100,000 deaths in various forms occur each year due to the effects of alcohol, half of them the result of injuries related to alcohol. According to a recent special report prepared for the United States Congress by the National Institute on Alcohol Abuse and Alcoholism, the cost of alcoholism to the nation is an estimated $185 billion annually. It's also estimated that one in four children is exposed to the ill effects of alcoholism.[18]

Homelessness and joblessness related to alcoholism are a major scourge of modern society. Do homelessness and joblessness cause alcoholism, or does alcoholism cause homelessness and joblessness? The answer is neither. The cause lies not in alcohol and not in a person's social circumstances, but in their brain. For this reason, brain training is especially effective with alcoholics. Hundreds of individuals have experienced brain training and become clean and sober, and they remain clean and sober years later.

Though numerous studies have been completed on Twelve Step programs, it's thought that only about twelve percent who enter a Twelve Step program are successful, in that they complete the steps and become clean and sober for life. It just so happens that, when we assess the brain of alcoholics, about twelve percent of those who are alcoholics are identified as likely to be genetically prone to addiction. Is it coincidental that this percentage is so similar to the percentage of people who are successful in Twelve Step programs? The same pattern persists in people who have been in AA for many years. This seems to indicate that people who appear to have a genetic propensity for alcoholism are the ones most likely to be successful in a Twelve Step program.[19]

Studying brain assessments reveals that others who train their brain to alleviate addiction fall into one of two categories. About eighty percent of them are suffering from internal anxiety for which they use alcohol as a sedative. Additionally, about eight percent suffer from situational anxiety and a fallacious belief system that causes them to habitually use alcohol as a sedative.

Alcoholics with internal anxiety are driven to quiet their high level of anxiety by using alcohol. A Twelve Step program can help such individuals create a basis for support, but it may not help them therapeutically as much as Cognitive Therapy or a Rational Emotive-based program. In fact, working the Twelve Steps alone without other therapeutic endeavors may cause the internal anxiety such individuals experience to increase. Anxiety can manifest in many different forms, like insomnia and night terrors, tremors, compulsive movement, inability to listen, attention deficit disorder, hyperactivity disorder, and phobias.

Those who have situational anxiety and a fallacious belief system tend to habitually self-medicate in an attempt to ease the pain of what they believe is a flaw in their being. Rather than face their mistaken belief about themselves, they choose to deaden their thinking altogether with medication, and often alcohol is their medication of choice.

If individuals don't have an addictive personality yet use alcohol to harmful excess, in most cases they are still unable to simply stop drinking. In this way they are no different from smokers. Most people who smoke don't really want to smoke. They even try to quit at some point but find they can't. This is because nicotine is a very effective drug. It picks you up when you are down, and it levels you off when you are up too high. In addition, it's readily available.

The answer for all who suffer from anxiety, whether they alleviate or reduce their suffering with alcohol, tobacco, or other drugs, is to balance their brain so the need for sedation disappears or is significantly reduced. In other words, brain training helps both those who benefit from Twelve Step programs and those who would benefit more from other programs or individual therapies. Although brain training may not be *the* answer to addiction for everyone, it's a part of the answer and can propel any addiction program or therapy to far greater success ratios at a much accelerated pace.

A Remarkable Experiment with Drug Addiction

In August 2005, in Prescott, Arizona, an enlightened drug court judge and a director in the probation department took a bold step and allowed nine county jail probationers to enter a program of brain training. These probationers averaged thirty-three years of age, had an average of seven convictions, had been drug addicts an average of thirteen years, and had an average of twelve arrests. All used methamphetamines, together with other substances including crack, cocaine, heroin, ecstasy, marijuana, alcohol, and tobacco.

Two of these were women in their last trimester of pregnancy, and both had used methamphetamines during the first trimester, which is extremely dangerous for a fetus. If a woman uses methamphetamines repeatedly in her first trimester, there is a high probability that the infant will be born in distress and face many risks. Both babies were born distress-free and healthy.

Among the four female probationers was a forty-four-year-old named Iris. Her mother, who was abusive, was continually in and out of mental institutions. Her father, who was both complacent and timid, subscribed to the philosophy of "never rock the boat." Not only could he not keep a job, he cowered before his violent wife. Iris grew up the second of four children, all of whom ended up as alcoholics and drug addicts.

Iris started drinking as a teenager, dropped out of high school to have her first child, and married the child's father, an alcoholic. After the couple had a second daughter, they drank their way to homelessness and eventual divorce. Without child support, Iris had to work three jobs to raise her girls, all the while suffering from depression. Iris' life was now so hard and so without hope, she turned to drugs for solace.

When Iris again married, it was to a methamphetamine addict. She too became an addict, and together they became the town's drug dealers. After their son was born, he and their two daughters were taken away by the state, but even now Iris couldn't break her drug habit. Methamphetamines and alcohol became her life, and she ended up on the street. Soon she was in jail. Not yet twenty-six years old, she had no teeth, weighed only ninety pounds, and was in extremely poor health.

A brighter episode of eleven months followed as a result of a women's drug program. But when she once more started to use, she ended up back in jail with a ninety-day sentence for misusing an elderly woman's credit cards. Five days after her release, she was back in jail again. It was only because a generous friend bailed her out and paid for an attorney that she came before an enlightened judge, who remanded her to a series of brain training sessions.

As Iris pulled herself back together in response to training her brain, for a time she was consumed with guilt over the waste of her life. For over thirty years she had cried herself to sleep, feeling helpless, worthless, and stupid—and now she realized it may all have been avoidable.

Several years later, Iris is now employed, clean and sober, and has her young son with her again. Though she doesn't understand how brain training works, she is clear about what it can accomplish. It gave her balanced judgment, clarity, and a steadiness she had not experienced before. This provided her with a foundation on which to rebuild her life. She is now happy, healthy, and productive.

Iris' proclivity for addiction was a true disability, tantamount to a birth defect, because she was raised lacking the basic tools needed to build a meaningful life. She grew up in despair and hopelessness, without any kind of experience of what a stable life looks like. But with brain training, she gained the focus needed to move out of the cycle of abuse and into the life she was born to live.

Iris was just one of nine probationers who, in this experiment in the summer of 2005, was given the option of brain training as part of the probation rehabilitation program. Two of the probationers have re-offended. All seven of the others are on a new path. Such is the transformative power of a brain that's balanced and in harmony. A balanced brain will self-regulate the body, the emotions, cognitive processing, and the spiritual life of the individual. The result is a balanced life that is productive and free from chains of addiction and antisocial behavior.

My experience has been that nine out of ten methamphetamine addicts can overcome their urge to use in three days of brain training, which seems impossible to conventional detoxification approaches—and they can stay clean forever with a total of twenty to thirty sessions when this effort is coupled with an effective substance abuse treatment program.

Brain training is also effective for addressing other forms of addiction such as recreational drugs, prescription drugs, sex, gambling, or shopping. So far, over six hundred people who have been addicted to substances, sex, gambling, or spending have seen their lives changed by training their brain. In each case, their brain assessment revealed a severe imbalance. But once balance was restored to the brain, the brain pattern that led them to seek balance in the form of a pathology was no longer needed. Things changed. Because they removed their *need* for their addiction, the addiction simply fell away, and they were free to follow their Twelve Step or addiction abatement program successfully.

18

Here's to Your Health!

Our culture has taught us to see illness from a diagnostic standpoint. We want an expert to tell us, "This is what's wrong with you."

We've all been taught that if we don't feel good or experience a health issue, we need a diagnosis. The diagnosis generally results from focusing on smaller and smaller elements of the problem, in the belief that a process of reductionism will provide the clearest understanding of the cause. Once the diagnosis has been figured out, we apply a particular treatment. However, a treatment directed at the smallest aspects of our illness may not have anything to do with the real cause of the disease and consequently can't furnish a lasting solution. Treating symptoms doesn't get at the cause.

The body of knowledge developing around quantum mechanics points us in a different direction. In fact, a quantum approach is somewhat foreign to both allopathic medicine and to clinical psychology. In these disciplines, the drive is to diagnose.

When it comes to helping people restore a state of wholeness, a quantum understanding of reality is far more helpful than a Newtonian worldview. Even though our knowledge of quantum physics is in many ways extremely theoretical, which makes it difficult to pin down (unlike Newtonian physics where you can measure things exactly), this growing body of knowledge has much to teach us because it shows us that the discrete, separate, independent "causes" we ascribe to illness are not necessarily what's really happening with respect to people's health. They are symptoms, not the *dis-ease* itself. The real cause is likely much more complex, and to one degree or another always involves the brain.

Because it is based in a quantum view of reality, brain training takes a different approach from diagnosing. If it's the case that balancing the brain affects the body beneficially, the reverse is also true. An unbalanced brain has a deleterious effect on our physical body, as well as on our psychological, emotional, and spiritual well-being. Though we often don't see the damaging effect of an unbalanced brain on our health right away—and, in fact, a person may go years without seeing the effect of an imbalance—at some point our health begins to deteriorate in an obvious manner.

The beauty of brain training is that it doesn't make any difference what the cause of an illness is. Brain training balances the neural network, harmonizing the brain's neighborhoods, and doesn't deal with one aspect of the system at a time or with a diagnosed disorder as a doctor would need to do. To discover the origin of a symptom can require an extremely complex and time-consuming investigation, but it's not necessary to know how symptoms are generated. By training the brain, all of the body's systems are helped to function more efficiently.

Instead of trying to diagnose what's going wrong in the body, all that brain training attempts to accomplish is to allow the brain to see itself in its optimized state. In fact, when you train your brain, you don't focus on what's wrong with you at all. Brain training really has no interest in what's wrong. Although brain training uses protocols that can have an effect on many pathologies, its purpose isn't to address a particular pathology. Rather, it's intended to create a basic balance and harmony between the various regions of the brain. When the brain is optimized, all of the bodily systems it regulates function better. If something has gone wrong in the body, by restoring a state of homeostasis we have a better chance of healing, because a balanced brain then seeks to bring the rest of the organism's biological, psychological, and emotional systems into balance.

In other words, the brain heals from inside out, which helps the body it regulates to also heal from inside out.

The Healing Power of a Balanced Brain

A balanced brain creates an environment in which our bodily functions are able to perform optimally. As with our mental well-being, it furnishes us with a level playing field. For instance, becoming balanced establishes a context in which cholesterol can fall into the normal range if we follow healthy practices that encourage beneficial cholesterol levels. Sometimes, even dramatic changes occur and the physical manifestation of *dis-ease* falls away completely.

There is nothing new about this phenomenon. From the beginning of recorded time there have been cases of what are often referred to as "miracles," whereby a cure happens spontaneously. Such cases number in the tens of thousands. When a person's internal state changes—when the energy pattern in the brain alters—it can result in a physical healing. In response to some kind of stimulus, whether subtle or more direct, the individual's brain pattern changes. As the brain is brought back into balance, the body responds accordingly.

How dramatically the brain affects the body can be seen from yogis in the East who have trained themselves to profoundly affect their body metabolism, slowing their heart rate and lowering their blood pressure. If we practice enough, we can all learn to change our heart rate and blood pressure.

Once the brain is functioning in an optimized state, it can't help but facilitate an improvement in physical health. Still, no matter how in balance the brain is, it can't compensate for eating a poor diet and failing to exercise and get adequate sleep. It just furnishes the context for the body to function at an optimal level when we do all the other things we need to do to be healthy.

In some cases, brain training puts the icing on the cake for a person recovering from a less than optimum condition. For instance, a man was experiencing erratic blood pressure readings. In the wake of an extremely stressful situation created by a natural disaster, this person found the base level of his blood pressure increased considerably. The most serious feature of this increase was that, at any given moment, his pressure would begin climbing out of control, which on more than one occasion sent him to the emergency room. Readings such as 248/136 were being reached in minutes, requiring immediate medical intervention. While medication could bring these levels under control to some degree, it couldn't cure the periodic extreme spiking.

It so happened that this person began brain training at this time. For most people, blood pressure normalizes soon after they begin training their brain. But in this particular case, no improvement was observed. However, a few weeks later, the individual began a weight loss protocol that employs the injectable hormone hCG (human chorionic gonadotrophin). Within two weeks, his blood pressure was greatly reduced, with no more spikes to dangerous levels. At this point, he returned for a further series of brain training sessions. Following the very first session, his pressure dropped to a stunningly healthy reading. The administering of hCG induced a change, which brain training was then able to capitalize on. After ceasing hCG injections, the individual's blood pressure remained healthy.

The brain has a tendency to want to balance itself even when it's stuck in an unbalanced state. As a result of injecting the hormone hCG, this individual's brain was given an opportunity to experience hormone levels that are conducive to normal blood pressure. Once his brain saw its ability to function with a more normal pressure, the additional brain training intensified his brain's new vision of itself, further improving the client's blood pressure readings.

How does training the brain improve blood pressure? Balancing the brain affects the nervous system, which in many cases drives hypertension. Throughout the day, hormonal changes occur in the body. These, coupled with tiredness at certain times of the day, may be reflected in a fluctuation in blood pressure. Imagine carrying a thirty-pound weight strapped to your waist and walking around all day doing a variety of activities. At some point you are likely to become really tired and have to push yourself to keep going. To do this, you begin to constrict your body. This tightening is the hypertension we experience. For most people with hypertension, brain training brings an immediate improvement as the brain moves into greater balance.

The warden of a medium security correctional facility had been abducted a few years before he tried brain training. During the abduction, inmates attempted to stab him to death as the correctional officers stormed the cellblock to free him. He survived, but then the trauma was compounded with the death of his father and a terrible car accident only months after his abduction. These horrific experiences left his autonomic nervous system completely out of balance, which resulted in high blood pressure—a reading of 180 over 120 even with medication—and also heart arrhythmia. As a dedicated professional, this courageous man began brain training to prove to his inmates, who were being offered the opportunity to train their brain, that it wasn't brain washing, electric shock treatment, or some other kind of invasive control of their behavior. The warden's courage brought great rewards. His blood pressure immediately fell into the normal range and his arrhythmia evaporated, a state that persisted without the need of medication. Additionally, the people who work with him, together with his family, have noted how much calmer and more focused he is—and, particularly, how much more fun and caring he has become.

The phenomenon is akin to when a baby is born addicted to methamphetamine because the mother has been on drugs. Such babies are often premature, underweight, and somewhat malnourished. I suspect the retarded physical development of the child results from the severely stressed state of its brain.

Even though tens or even hundreds of thousands of dollars of care are required to sustain the life of a methamphetamine child, the stress the child has endured doesn't go away by itself. On the contrary, it continues to restrict the child's ability to develop normally. Energy that should be directed toward healthy growth is instead directed to keeping the child in a continuous mode of fight-or-flight. In such a state, insecurity drives the child's every behavior, resulting in a complete inability to trust, coupled with frequent emotional outbursts. These little brains need lots of tender loving care, augmented with brain training, to help them grow into productive, healthy, happy people.

Slowing the Aging Process

Is it possible to slow the aging process through brain training? If we take a cross section of humanity, it's immediately apparent that people's appearance and vitality at any given age varies greatly. There are individuals who look extremely young for their age, while others don't seem to age well at all. Our observation from seeing thousands of people train their brain is that when someone's brain begins to process in a balanced way, they tend not to appear as old as their years say they are. Their eyes turn up a bit, their skin is somewhat renewed, wrinkles either vanish or blend to create a wise, sophisticated look, and sexual functioning is renewed.

In each of us, there's a program running that says it's time to start winding down. For men it happens at around forty, and for women about ten years later, coinciding with menopause. Often after age forty the person becomes unglued, experiencing what we call a midlife crisis. It's also after forty that people tend to start having problems reading a restaurant menu without glasses because their eyes don't focus as they once did.

A second major time of physical decline occurs after the age of sixty. In women, there's a high occurrence of breast and uterine cancer at this time of life. In men, erectile dysfunction often occurs, while prostate cancer affects a high percentage of males over fifty. According to the American College of Physicians, autopsy results show that more than half of men over the age of fifty have prostate cancer. Clinically, about 17% of men over age fifty are diagnosed with prostate cancer. Prostate cancer is the second-leading cause of cancer death in men, behind lung cancer.[20] In fact, prostate cancer happens at four times the rate of breast cancer and is the second biggest killer of men.[21]

Brain training can often help in such cases. For example, seven men with elevated PSA scores who subsequently trained their brain all found themselves returning to the normal range of PSA. This is likely because, with the brain, we are talking about the central processing unit for the body, which runs our autonomic nervous system and controls every feature of our bodily organs. When the brain is balanced, all of the body's organs work more effectively, blood flows more freely, and toxins are eliminated more readily. Many men with erectile dysfunction find they attain a natural erection once their brain is in balance. Their level of enjoyment also increases as the sexual organs more easily engorge with blood. Women also lubricate more readily. When a male's erectile dysfunction diminishes, or a female's vaginal dryness becomes less of a problem, both enjoy sex more fully and with less stress.

It's important at any age to feel we are attractive, desirable, and a sexual being. If a male experiences erectile dysfunction, but for health reasons such as hypertension can't use something like Viagra or a natural approach such as the herb yohimbe, he might become depressed. Is the depression causing erectile dysfunction, or is erectile dysfunction triggering the depression?

Consider the case of a person who tells their physician, "I'm depressed and my libido is low." The health practitioner or psychiatrist tries to solve the person's depression with a prescription because, from a medical standpoint, the problem is that the patient has too much of one chemical and too little of another. But this chemical change might not bring the brain back into balance. "We'll solve your depression, and that will solve your erectile dysfunction" is something a health professional cannot promise. The simple fact is, not only does exercise often work better than antidepressants in overcoming depression, exercise also enhances sexual functioning. When we balance our brain, balance our diet, and get a moderate amount of exercise, we are likely to experience a far greater degree of contentment in every area of our life.

A Surprising Discovery

As we saw in an earlier chapter, most people in western culture have overactive high frequency brain patterns, which is a very fast brain state. The energy reservoir of the brain is mostly depleted, which indicates a lack of reserve. It's like the moving parts of an engine working rapidly without oil. This has a negative impact on wellness.

In the case of Alzheimer's or dementia, you would think you would see a great many quiet areas in the brain, as well as in cases of chronic fibromyalgia, chronic fatigue, and Epstein Barr. Often it's just the opposite. You'd think you'd want to increase brain activity. The reality is that if activity decreases, and the client balances and harmonizes the brain patterns, the brain has the opportunity to heal itself. If somebody is using medication to sustain themselves while training their brain, it might take longer. This is because, although the individual receives the same effect from a brain training session, the effect may not last as long in the presence of medication. Still, the brain will work to heal itself in the presence of most medications over time.

Incidentally, a helpful therapy for Alzheimer's is to change as many things as possible for the patient. If they generally get up on one side of the bed, have them get up on the other. If they sit at the head of the table, have them sit at the side. Have them eat different things for breakfast each day. Change the newspaper they read.

Take them on a different route for their walk and encourage brushing their teeth with the other hand. By changing as many things as possible, the individual sustains brain flexibility, which keeps the neural patterns in better shape.

Recall that the protocols used to train the brain evolved using the original brain assessments of two Buddhist monks. Since then, we have assimilated information from thousands of brain assessments to fine-tune the original algorithms. Honing the algorithms continues as the brain assessments of more and more clients are examined.

As the relevance of the differences between individuals became intelligible, it was possible to include more and more information in the training protocols. This is useful because a person with a particular pathology might exhibit one brain pattern, whereas someone with the same pathology might manifest a quite different pattern. As noted earlier, people with depression exhibit over a dozen patterns. The same is true for panic attacks and ADHD. In fact, more than one pattern of imbalance is evident for virtually all of the pathologies observed.

Brain Training Helps You Take Charge of Physical Pain

Another area of health in which brain training can be immensely valuable is pain management. It can help because pain isn't simply a local issue in the body but involves the brain.

If you have a shower with two shower heads in the ceiling, but you live alone and get into a habit over a long period of time of only using one of the two heads, it never occurs to you that the other head even exists. In due course, the showerhead you use all the time will start dripping from excess use.

Think about this in terms of the signals going from your left and right hands up your arms to your brain. Generally, both hands will send a comparable number of messages to the brain, unless you are particularly using one hand for an activity such as writing. However, in an attempt to hammer a nail, you accidentally hit a finger on your left hand. In such a situation, your left hand sends many times more signals to your brain than your right hand because it's crying out for attention. The signals to the brain become lopsided—just like running only one showerhead.

When the brain receives repeated messages from a part of the body that's in pain, it causes the brain to become hyper-vigilant where this region of the body is concerned. Even as it receives many more signals from the painful spot, it also fires signals to this spot as if to ask, "Are you all right? Are you sure you are all right?" The result is that a feedback loop is established.

If we hurt a finger by hammering it, we are extra careful not to bump it. Yet, somehow, despite our attempts to protect it, such a finger tends to get bumped—and when it does, it hurts inordinately. Why is this?

A small bump sends a lot of signals indicating pain. This causes the motor signal that controls movement to become slightly imbalanced because the sensory signal is being used so much more. This imbalance gives us less control over a finger, even though we are trying our utmost to protect it. It's akin to a parent hovering over a child all the time, to the point the child becomes almost incapable of taking care of itself. Just as a child whose parent hovers tends to experience diminished competence, a finger that's hurt isn't so easy to control and tends to get bumped!

It's helpful to know that a finger is sore. But when the body sends signals back to the brain so frequently that the brain becomes unbalanced, the brain begins to expect problems. Consequently, usually insignificant issues now loom large. In this situation, a small bump to an already-hurting finger will register with a much higher intensity of pain.

In such a situation, the brain has a tendency to rebalance itself, but often we don't allow this to happen. Instead, we use painkillers to mitigate the pain. The messages from the pain keep coming back to the brain, but they aren't received as strongly. When the messages don't register as they should, the number of messages increases. This is what leads to a condition of chronic pain. We find ourselves in a Catch 22. The longer we use a painkiller, the greater the quantity of medication required to produce the same amount of relief. In due course, the painkiller may not work at all.

If a person takes steps to balance their brain, a similar mitigation of pain is often experienced. On a scale of one to ten, with ten being the most severe, pain generally moves from a level of eight or nine to five or six. By diminishing pain, brain training lessens the hold chronic pain has on us so we can better enjoy our life.

Inflammation is also in part the result of an imbalance in the brain. The imbalance isn't the direct cause. Usually, a trauma shifts the autonomic nervous system into a state of imbalance, and this results in inflammation. Conditions like rheumatoid arthritis only occur because there is underlying inflammation. Like most other chronic pain, such conditions are often improved simply by balancing the brain.

When inflammation manifests as an aspect of a disease, it poses a question concerning the origin of the disease. Was the disease caused by a breakdown of the diseased tissue or organ? Or was it caused because the brain was severely imbalanced, which was then duplicated in an imbalance of the physiology?

In the case of childbirth pain, you might think that extreme pain is simply a given. Yet there are women who experience only minimal pain compared with others who are in agony. Why?

Society pushes women to see themselves as sexual objects. Consequently, when they are expecting a child, many women tend to see themselves as overweight and unattractive. This can contribute to becoming uptight, which has a tightening effect on the body's musculature. As the breasts enlarge and the abdomen swells to allow the fetus to grow, what's required is elasticity. Elasticity is also required for the pelvic region during delivery. The less flexible the female musculature is, the more pain the woman experiences. The more relaxed and flexible a woman's body is, the easier the birth process. When the brain is balanced, people are automatically more relaxed. Brain training enables a woman to relax, which is beneficial for both the growth of the baby and the woman's enjoyment of her pregnancy. Childbirth proceeds more smoothly when the body isn't constricted.

Put yourself in a heavy stress situation. All of us have areas where stress tends to reside—our neck, our shoulders, or our back. How relaxed we are is crucial. Relaxation facilitates a full range of motion. New information about stretching suggests we shouldn't stretch more than in short bursts of two seconds at a time because the muscle responds by tightening if we stretch for more than a few seconds.[22]

Many forms of pain are eased when a person's brain is in balance. Sharp pain from an injury and subsequent raw nerve is lessened. Dull, throbbing pain that may have to do with a post-surgical condition improves. Tired, achy pain often related to stress and the vulnerability of a specific region of the body is eased.

When I had a frozen shoulder all those years I was suffering from post-traumatic stress disorder, there was a limited mechanical problem and a major brain imbalance. Once the initial injury healed, I should have been able to move the shoulder freely. However, the injury was related to a brain imbalance. As I stated earlier, once I solved the brain imbalance, I was able to work with a trainer and pretty soon could use my shoulder fully.

The brain is not only a player in our health, but *the* central player. For this reason, it's my belief that brain training will be considered for inclusion alongside most, if not all, of the healing modalities as time progresses.

19

Traumatic Brain Injury

A TRAUMATIC BRAIN INJURY, whether from an external or internal source, produces a severe imbalance in brainwave energy. The injury can be caused by something as simple as a blow to the head. Often the effects are greatest immediately following the injury.

The newly injured brain suffers damage from swelling and a form of bruising known as a contusion. Due to the malfunctioning of the brain environment caused by the blow, it may require many weeks before the extent of the damage can be determined. Age is a component of the prognosis. Children often have more brain flexibility and therefore can progress more rapidly than adults with similar damage.

Damage of this kind can render a person unconscious, leaving them in a coma. Others are conscious but not aware. In some cases, a multitude of cognitive problems follow the initial injury, including difficulty with concentration and organizing thoughts, becoming easily confused, being forgetful, having difficulty learning new information, and finding it hard to solve problems, make decisions, or plan anything. Varying degrees of difficulty with language can result from a trauma of this kind, including poor sentence formation, difficulty with appropriate word detection, lengthy or faulty descriptions or explanations, stuttering, and problems utilizing the voice to demonstrate emotional intensity. While some cannot express themselves, others have difficulty understanding language, especially if it's part of a joke, a sarcastic remark, or an adage. Difficulties with reading and writing are also common. In some cases there's a loss of awareness of social boundaries and social skills, making social situations difficult for the individual.

Individuals with a traumatic brain injury can easily become frustrated due to the lack of control they experience. Impaired motor skills, trouble expressing themselves, and difficulty with understanding things can cause severe frustration, which emerges as anger and rage. Repeated outbursts tend to establish patterns of behavior not only in the individual suffering from a brain injury, but also among family and friends who live around the individual. If symptoms persist beyond six weeks, it may be helpful for the family unit to undergo brain training in order to create new patterns of social interaction.

A traumatic brain injury leaves an imbalance in the autonomic nervous system. With severe stress, particularly at the time of injury, the brain shifts into either a freeze response or a fight-flight response. The freeze state is associated with the shunting of blood from muscles to organs in the body core. The racing heart slows to a crawl, blood pressure drops, and tense muscles collapse and become still. Additionally, memory access and storage are impaired, resulting in some degree of amnesia.

If a freeze state remains dominant after a traumatic brain injury, the result can be depression, dizziness or lightheadedness, decreased clarity of thought, confusion, difficulty organizing thoughts, fatigue, bowel problems, a low heart rate, and peripheral neuropathy (damage to the network that transmits information from the central nervous system to every other part of the body).

If a fight-or-flight state is dominant, a greater alertness, increased energy, and greater muscle strength are experienced. Blood pressure and heart rate increase, and pupils dilate to let more light into the eyes in order to increase visual acuity. This can result in hyper-vigilance, nervousness, panic attacks, anxiety, fear and paranoia, poor sleep, shakiness and heart palpitations, stroke, heart attack, heart disease, cold hands and feet, and headaches.

The Devastating Effect of Serious Brain Imbalance

If either the parasympathetic or sympathetic nervous systems become totally dominant in key areas of the brain as a result of trauma, problems with the digestive tract are inevitable.

Take the case of Janet, who was hit by a car and suffered a broken back from the accident, necessitating spinal surgery. Because no one recognized at the time that an accident of this kind has a devastating effect on the brain, triggering acute autonomic nervous system imbalance, this nineteen-year-old's life became a living hell.

Two years after the accident, Janet began developing a series of health difficulties, focused around digestion, which led to twenty years of surgeries and countless periods of time in hospitals.

Janet's difficulties started with colitis, which became increasingly problematic, ultimately leading to the removal of her colon.

After undergoing so many surgeries and so much time in the hospital, Janet's immune system was all but wrecked. She had reached her limit both physically and emotionally and could take no more. She decided it was time to quit all treatment and simply allow the chips to fall where they may.

At the initial conference, Janet's family were present and spelled out how dire the situation had become. They expressed their daughter's deep need either to be well or to move beyond this life.

It was made clear that the purpose of brain training isn't to make people well—that keeping people alive isn't the task of brain training. However, balancing and harmonizing brain patterns could help a person walk through the threshold of death in such a manner that they could feel and be who they are throughout the dying process, instead of their identity being hijacked by the health problems and physical torment that encompass them.

Janet and her family accepted the inevitability of death. For the last four years especially, Janet's life had been devastating. For instance, she practically slept in the bathroom—at least, to the extent she was able to sleep, which was usually no more than dozing off for around ten minutes at a time. She couldn't relax watching a movie because she couldn't sit for much more than ten minutes. Her life was oriented around being close to a bathroom, to the point she could only go to a store if it was a short drive and she knew where the bathroom was. In such a state, life seemed to Janet to no longer have a purpose.

When brain training began, the huge energy differences in all the lobes of the brain started to change, and for the first time in twenty years Janet sat and watched a movie with her family, then slept for five and a half hours. Consequently, Janet found herself spontaneously moving back from the door to death and into a re-engagement of life. I believe that this young woman will use her journey to somehow become an important person on the planet, and her better-balanced brain will be the enabler of that positive life action.

The Power to Rise Above Our Limitations

Mentally handicapped from birth, which doctors say may have resulted from having to have a shunt inserted in her heart in the womb, causing brain damage due to lack of oxygen, in many ways Ruth was like a twelve-year-old in a thirty-year-old body.

Until Ruth trained her brain, her motor skills were compromised, and hence her movements were somewhat spastic. For instance, she couldn't ascend a flight of stairs by simply placing one foot ahead of the other in a fluid manner. Instead, she had to take a single step at a time, pausing after each step. Her speech was also a little difficult to follow.

In terms of her personality, Ruth was shy and reserved when interacting with people. She works in a beauty parlor helping the beauticians prepare their materials, arranging their work area, laying out everything they need. Before she began training her brain, she didn't interact much with the people she worked among but simply did her job. She rarely made eye contact and talked only minimally. Whenever she became even the least bit anxious, her skin reddened and she began sweating profusely. At home, her family found her to be cranky much of the time, and she preferred to spend time alone in her room rather than with everyone else.

After her first brain training intensive, Ruth was already a different person. Her smile lit up the room, and she became a chatterbox both at home and her place of work. People she didn't like now became people she spoke to instead of ignoring them.

Ruth's motor skills have also greatly improved, to the point that she flies up a flight of stairs. As a result, she has expressed a desire to take dance lessons. Because she is now able to retain three or four instructions at a time, whereas before training she could only remember the last instruction she was given, dancing becomes a real possibility for her. The ability to retain information also means she may be able to fulfill her dream of returning to school to learn computer skills. As she continues to train her brain, she finds herself more and more in charge of her life. Presently, she is training herself to be less scattered and absent-minded, which will help her pursue her goals.

Training a Brain in a Coma

A particularly striking example of recovery from a traumatic brain injury is that of Charlotte, a scientist, fluent in Spanish and English, with published scholarly books in both languages.

About a week after giving birth to triplets, Charlotte suffered a brain hemorrhage. It was thought she was only experiencing a headache and consequently signs of the hemorrhage weren't detected. In fact, Charlotte received medication for a headache and to help her sleep. The result was she didn't wake up the next morning.

When the family tried unsuccessfully to awaken Charlotte, she was taken to the hospital. There, doctors advised her family to allow her to remain comfortable due to the extent of the damage. Instead, the family insisted she have surgery to stop the bleeding happening in both sides of her brain. The surgery was successful, but the prognosis was that Charlotte would be a vegetable for the rest of her life. Her family was assured she would never come out of the coma and cessation of life support should be considered.

Charlotte's brother James had become a brain training licensee shortly before Charlotte's triplets were born. James was allowed to take a computer inside the hospital, where he conducted an assessment of his sister's brain. In the assessment process, a person is asked to perform a series of simple but specific mental tasks. The tasks are designed to activate the lobes that are being assessed. Of course, Charlotte wasn't able to open her eyes at all. Nor was she able to answer the questions and perform the tasks.

James' approach was to assume that Charlotte could hear the instructions she was being given, even though she couldn't speak, couldn't open her eyes, and couldn't communicate in any other way. James told his sister, "I know you are unable to respond, so I will respond for you, and you do the task along with me in your mind."

In one of the tasks, a client repeats numbers with their eyes open. James carried this exercise out in both the role of trainer and client. For instance, he might have called out the numbers one, seven, ten, nine, six, four, and eleven. Instead of Charlotte repeating the numbers, James repeated them for her.

When the brain assessment data was examined, it was apparent that Charlotte's brain patterns had altered dramatically from the time when she was supposed to be at rest to the time when she was supposed to have her eyes open at task. Yet all the while, Charlotte was in a coma!

When Charlotte didn't emerge from the coma, the doctors concluded it was impossible for her to recover because there simply were no biological markers reflecting the kind of neural activity that would lead to consciousness and full ability to sustain life. But during the assessment, the EEG-based assessment data did in fact change distinctly, and the trainer could observe the difference from one minute to the next. There was no doubt at all that Charlotte could hear and follow what was being said to her. Even if she didn't follow and hear cognitively, she was responding with an energy pattern that could pick up on the information and follow it at some level. The results weren't imaginary; they were measurable in pure scientific terms.

When James pointed out the brain activity to the hospital, they allowed him to begin training Charlotte in her hospital room, though they were convinced he was wasting his time. In fact, whenever he arrived with his computer to train his sister, they referred to him as "Crazy James and the brain machine."

Within six weeks, Charlotte opened her eyes. A year later, she is at home, able to walk though still with many issues for ongoing physical therapy, and able to understand and talk in both Spanish and English like she could before her brain hemorrhage. Although she has a long way to go for there to be a full recovery, the distance she has journeyed is light years compared with being in a coma. There may be some areas in which she will not have full functionality, while in other aspects of life she may be able to function even more effectively.

The element that made the difference was the courage of the family.

More money is expended on brain disease and brain injury—which includes such conditions as stroke, Alzheimer's, and dementia—than on all other diseases put together.[23] Traumatic brain injury and brain diseases are devastating. But even some of the worst cases are not necessarily beyond the help brain training can provide when it is used with current treatments and therapies.

20

You Are Changing Yourself

AFTER A FEW SESSIONS OF TRAINING THEIR BRAIN, people occasionally remark, "I don't feel any different, so I don't think it's working."

A classic example of this is a man with Parkinson's disease who was using a combination of a wheelchair and a walker and couldn't speak well. The training didn't seem to be making any difference to any of his conditions.

Then, two weeks after he experienced ten sessions of training, he got up one morning, walked into the kitchen without either his wheelchair or walker, and began making coffee. When his wife entered the room, he struck up a conversation with her as if nothing extraordinary were going on.

"Oh, my God!" his wife exclaimed. "Oh, my God!"

The husband was totally unaware of the dramatic change that

had taken place in his condition. What he was doing seemed completely normal to him. His story isn't unique. There's often a remarkable spin-off from brain training in individuals with degenerative problems—although the process is apt to work slowly, with many of the deeper changes coming about gradually. Brain training is not yet known to sustain such change in most clients with degenerative diseases, but will likely be one of the tools used to promote healing of such diseases.

Like the man with Parkinson's, individuals are sometimes dramatically changed, yet initially they don't recognize how great the change is because it's such an integral part of their sense of themselves. Everyone around them can see they are different, but they can't detect the differences. Even if they feel better, the shifts they experience are so organic to the brain that the way they now feel and act seems perfectly natural to them, as if they had always been this way. In fact, it is natural—the way we were meant to be.

One reason change feels so natural is that when a person is in the midst of most brain imbalances that manifest in pathology, the brain is functioning automatically. Consequently, the person may not be aware they are experiencing an imbalance. It's not as if they were thinking in ways that cause their brain to be unbalanced, and they certainly aren't willing it to function with an imbalance. So when the brain is trained to regain its balance, it tends to work automatically just as it did when it was in a state of imbalance, which means the individual may be unaware a change has occurred. Only as the person gains greater distance from the time of the change do they see the difference in their behavior and realize they are functioning with a more balanced brain.

If you aren't immediately aware of changes, don't be disheartened. Eventually, the internal realization of the differences brain training brings about almost always catches up with the improvement in our functioning and behavior. In the meantime, pay attention to the details of your life, where you are likely to witness clear indications the process is working. As an example, the corners of a woman's eyes were down when she came for training. But following training, the corners were up and she looked bright and alive. We also notice that a person's eyes often sparkle—they just look so much more *present.*

The number of sessions required to achieve brain homeostasis varies from one client to the next, and homeostasis often comes about in phases. Certain changes are observed first, then later other improvements are noticed. It's like layers of an onion. We deal with one problem, then another underneath comes into view.

Earlier, we met former U.S. Marine Mick Patrick DeBriwere. Like that of so many, his experience in response to training his brain was a greater ability to be present. He comments, "There is a somatic truth"—he's talking about an experience that can be felt in the body—"in this brain training process that's self-evident and doesn't require the rigor of conceptualization. I accept the gift as it is. Being content with the Now would be considered the polar opposite of the hyper-vigilant anxiety that accompanies post-traumatic stress disorder. Some of the unbidden fear that frequently intrudes on my daily existence seems to have been a bit abated."

Mick felt like he actually inhabited his body for a change. This is one of the effects of training the brain. Bodily functions are governed by the brain, so when the brain is in balance, we feel in harmony with our physical makeup. We are at home in our body at last.

Mick's sense of being present in his body soon spilled over into his thoughts and feelings. He explains, "I feel a quieting of the rapid-fire sub-vocalizations that generally accompany me throughout my waking hours. And my wife reports that I don't seem to have the customary buildup to a jet stream of activity. She says she has witnessed me sitting quietly completing projects without distracting myself. She also states that my behavior and communications are less defensive, and that I am smiling more. I guess I cannot ask for more than these fine new attributes. And all I had to do was sit still for ten sessions with trainers who exuded a loving aura. Clearly, a poor man's heaven!"

Once a person is at home in their body and at peace with their thoughts, being truly engaged in the everyday tasks of life comes easier. As Mick reports, "I have noticed a clarity in internal dialogue, resulting in more ease in focusing."

It's truly wonderful when a man disabled by Parkinson's walks into the kitchen without a wheelchair or walker and begins fixing coffee for his wife. It's thrilling when physical wellness flows from training the brain. But the greater miracle is when we are so changed inside that, even if we don't see external manifestations of the change, we nevertheless lead a life of greater contentment, joy, and love.

Obvious to Everyone but Us!

Try an experiment. Sit in a chair, raise your right arm and your right foot, and turn both in a clockwise circular motion. It's quite easy to do.

Now turn your arm in the opposite, counterclockwise direction while keeping your foot moving in a clockwise direction. Invariably your foot will change direction too! But with time and practice, you can train your foot and your arm to move in opposite directions.

The brain automatically synchronizes the movement of the right foot with the movement of the right hand. If we thrust our right arm out to the right of our body with sufficient force, the brain causes the right leg to move to the right also in order to maintain our balance. Both actions are evidence of the automatic functioning of the brain.

Brain training is like learning to move your foot and your arm in circles independently. Homeostasis and severe imbalance are on opposite ends of the well-being continuum. Homeostasis is to imbalance what light is to a dark room. It's a foundation on which well-being is established, and the foundation of a building is often the phase of any construction that takes the most time and where for a while it can look like little is happening.

Take the case of a young man who appeared to be shy because he looked down a lot. In fact, his entire posture reflected an underlying feeling of inadequacy. It was little wonder he felt this way because he had been convicted of a crime that took a person's life. When this young man's brain was assessed, the parasympathetic side of his autonomic nervous system was running at two hundred percent above the sympathetic side! In only one training session, this imbalance changed dramatically. He looked better, his eyes were clearer, his head was no longer down but sat erect on his shoulders, and he walked in a way that was more alive.

The young man wasn't aware of the changes at first. It was only when he began hearing from others how different he was that he realized he really was different. "My family tells me I've changed tremendously," he reported. "I hear from people all the time, 'Son, you look good.' My teacher says, 'Wow, you are doing really well. You got an A– in English, whereas before you couldn't even speak clearly. Now you are writing in a clear form. Congratulations.'"

Positive feedback of this kind reinforces the changes the brain has made, fortifying the balance we have begun to achieve. It's as if the mind says to the brain, "This is a very good thing. You have served me well. Now I'm ready for the next stage of your development."

Sometimes we don't realize how much we have changed because the change allows memories to come up that involve emotional pain that's been etched deeply into us over the years, so it actually feels as if we are taking steps backwards for a time.

A case in point is a woman who accomplished such pleasing changes in her behavior that her boyfriend came to train as a result of the differences he saw in her. Subsequently, six of her friends also came to train. Yet the woman herself couldn't recognize how much she had changed! In fact, this woman questioned her trainer's ability because for a time she felt *worse*. It proved to be the darkness before the dawn, and the results were life-giving for her.

Why was this? The answer is that her feelings had been suppressed for years. When she suddenly began to really *feel* for the first time since she was young, it made her angry! The training had switched on a lot of repressed emotion she hadn't been aware of, which she now had to balance before she could experience the peace, joy, and love that was her natural state. With most modalities, this process would take months or even years. With brain training, the process usually takes only a few days.

When Change Is Slow

Training the brain involves developing new neural pathways, which ultimately result in behavior that's more conscious. Although this happens relatively quickly, it's a process that has to occur organically and can't be rushed.

If you undergo a series of brain training sessions and find yourself doing well and sleeping well, then two weeks later you seem to be less functional than you were when you completed training, don't let this discourage you. It doesn't mean the training isn't working.

If the training weren't working, you wouldn't have felt good in the first place. More training sessions will restore the new pathways to a position of dominance, and the advantages of training will be almost immediately experienced when training resumes.

In physics, for every force there's an equal but opposing force. The brain is subject to these same forces. A part of the brain resists change, and it resists it much more strongly if it can't discern that such a change would be safe and helpful. When we hold an intention for something good in our lives, we also sometimes experience doubt and even resistance to the good ever becoming a reality. If our resistance is equal in strength to our good intention, we get nowhere. Being persistent toward the good will always win eventually.

How awareness, courage, and persistence claim the victory every time can be seen in the case of Debbie. Before she began training her brain, she was plagued with an inability to stay focused. Her mind jumped from thought to thought so rapidly that she was unable to stay with any topic long enough to think it through. She was also unable to recall detail. In fact, her memory was so poor, the specifics of what happened even the previous day were lost to her, with only the vague outline of events remaining. As a consequence, she found herself constantly apologizing to friends and family for all the things they told her but that she didn't remember.

Debbie's inability to remember affected every aspect of her life, especially her performance in school and her relationships. It's extremely difficult to have a meaningful relationship with someone if they can't remember a thing you tell them. Not only did this make life extremely challenging for Debbie, she struggled with feelings of inferiority because of her constant failure to remember important information.

Although Debbie wished there was a way to improve her memory, she was skeptical when she first learned of brain training because her condition dated back to her earliest days and therefore seemed permanent. "I had learned to live my entire life with it," she explains, "and I just couldn't see reversing or fixing something so deeply entrenched in my head with a few sessions of training."

Then it occurred to Debbie that even a small improvement would be of huge benefit, so she mustered the courage to give it a go. The first couple of sessions were challenging for her. "I was left mentally exhausted," she recalls, "and with a headache." When friends and family saw her after the initial sessions, they all observed how tired, incoherent, dazed, and confused she seemed to be. But Debbie didn't give up.

As training continued, Debbie began to notice a change. When she awakened each morning, she felt more alert. For the first time, she sensed she had a measure of control over her thoughts. People around her remarked that she seemed more coherent. Debbie realized she was experiencing something she had never before experienced, a sensation that she was coming alive. "I felt like I was beginning to access the left side of my brain," she says. The video monitor displaying her brainwaves confirmed that both the left and right sides of her brain were now functioning in balance, whereas the left side had been largely inactive in her assessment.

By the end of training, Debbie was far more alert and enjoying a sense of mental clarity. She found herself relaxed, and her ability to retrieve information had greatly improved. For example, she could find the right words to express her thoughts and answer questions, and she was actually finishing her sentences. Instead of being bombarded by random thoughts, she was able to focus. Everyone could see she was handling stressful situations rationally at last. Faced with a difficulty, she was now able to problem-solve using previously learned information rather than simply reacting emotionally.

Roadblocks to Change

For change to happen, the brain must realize the change is safe. Even though the brain doesn't like to give up its pattern and therefore doesn't change readily, once it discerns that a new state isn't threatening, it spontaneously moves toward balance and harmony—toward homeostasis.

The brain's resistance can be heightened by a variety of external factors. For instance, the likelihood is that if a person is using certain medications, they will have a problem realizing change. Beta blockers and other like medication tend to relax how neurons fire, so that messages can't be carried as readily and training therefore doesn't happen as easily.

Alcohol also has a tendency to stop neural networks from expanding. People who train their brain are strongly discouraged from using alcohol for at least three weeks after they complete their training.

Speaking of the effects of alcohol on the brain, in the television series *Cheers*, Cliff explained to Norm that buffalo stay in a herd and only move as fast as the slowest buffalo. So, when the herd is attacked by predators and the buffalo run for their lives, the slowest members of the herd are left behind and become prey. Cliff reasoned that this is helpful to the herd as, with its slower members eliminated, the herd as a whole can move faster. Based on this, Cliff contended, alcohol destroys our slowest neurons, and therefore alcohol is actually good for the brain as it helps it move faster. The reasoning is hilarious, but of course far from the truth. Alcohol is a toxin. The reality is, if one even smells an alcoholic beverage by sniffing a glass or open bottle, the brain's activity immediately slows and undergoes change. This is adversarial to the intent of brain training, which aims to broaden and deepen neural activity, not restrict it.

Since brain training encourages the brain to stabilize itself, anything that has a tendency to change the activation pattern of the neural network is best deferred for a while. This gives the brain a chance to reach homeostasis. Cranial-sacral adjustments and chiropractic spinal manipulations are examples of protocols that alter brain patterns. It's important to suspend such treatments during brain training and for at least three weeks afterwards. Acupuncture, acupressure, and really deep tissue massage can also alter brain patterns, so their use is discouraged for a while too.

Anyone considering heavy chelation or detoxification would be wise to wait about three months after brain training before starting such treatments. Chelation is a process that loosens heavy metals so they pass out of the body through the liver and kidneys. It's important to be aware that the brain is the key player in the detoxification process and not to overload its capabilities. Since chelation releases heavy metals and toxins into the bloodstream, and the brain uses more blood when it's being trained, it's wise to keep the blood free of an overload of contaminants. For this reason, chelation may not be supportive during brain training. As a matter of fact, after training their brain, individuals with heavy metal toxicity have been known to spontaneously rid their body of these metals in the weeks and months following training, circumventing the need for some heavy chelation.

People can do three dozen chelation sessions and still find their heavy metal toxicity high. They can't flush it out. This is where brain training can help. Humans have a series of pipes in the body that facilitate a flow of bodily fluids. If we are in a state of imbalance, these pipes may not function optimally. If our sympathetic nervous system is high, the pipes tend to narrow. If our parasympathetic is high, they tend to be constricted in particular areas. As fluid flows through the pipes carrying heavy metal sediment, it slows where narrowed and backs up when there is constriction, which causes the sediment to drop out of the flow. When there is a balloon, the flow slows, and once again the sediment drops out. So, despite efforts to rid the body of toxicity by means of chelation, much of the heavy metal remains in the body. On the other hand, if a person alternates brain training with chelation, utilizing several rounds of each and keeping the different protocols about three months apart, the tubes are no longer constricted or narrowed and the heavy metals are flushed out of the body.

What about aromatherapy? A wide variety of aromas were tested over a six-month period to see whether a particular aroma might enhance brain training, but the benefit of all the aromas tested was negligible compared to brain training alone. Although many aromas appear to have a somewhat positive effect, how a particular aromatherapy will affect a given person seems to be unique to the individual. Until such time as there is sufficient data to determine which aromas help build beneficial brain patterns, it's wise to avoid aromatherapy when brain training. Similarly, how your office or home smells, and what perfume or cologne you wear, can be a factor in the effectiveness of training.

Why this is so can be seen from putting an onion in front of someone's nose. Whether the individual is happy or sad, asleep or awake, the onion will have an instant effect on them. They will jerk back. Even if they are asleep, they will react. Happy, sad, or sleeping, it makes no difference because the olfactory center in the brain has no filters, which means that smelling something produces an immediate response. In other words, olfactory has a direct influence on the brain.

It might seem strange that a particular scent could have such an impact on the brain's balance. Although the brain is robust, it's also a delicate instrument that can easily be thrown out of balance.

When we realize how sensitive the brain is, it's easy to understand how, if a person bumps their head, and the bump isn't even hard enough to leave a bruise but just for a second they experience a tinge of blurry vision, a slight adjustment occurs in their brain. Olfactory cues can cause a similar response.

Even when all of the factors that might cause resistance to transformation have been considered, some people appear to experience no effect from training their brain. Perhaps between ten and fifteen percent of the population don't seem to respond. There isn't sufficient data yet to know why this is. It's possible that, depending on the pathology, it will be necessary to combine brain training with another modality. Brain training was never intended to be a panacea.

What about maintenance? Should we obtain regular brain maintenance, just as we would with a car?

Especially in the beginning, as new neural networks are forming, it can be helpful to have the reinforcement of additional training. A brain pattern can shift quite quickly at times, but it may need support for a while until the new pattern is firmly established.

One woman likes to have one session of training a week to keep her in optimal condition. Her rationale is that it's better to pay for brain training than to pay a masseuse, as she feels more relaxed and sleeps better with brain training. Of course, a person could opt for both brain training and a massage! It's not difficult to understand why this person is so enthusiastic about training. When she started training, she was using a large number of medications. Her whole day was spent looking at her watch, following a schedule of medication. In twenty sessions, she was down to a reasonable number of prescriptions. Currently, she's down to two or three, and these only on an as-needed basis.

Helping the Healing and Self-realization Process

In November 2006, a fifty-two year old woman suffered a stroke that paralyzed her left arm and leg. Her progress in physical therapy was slow. In order to cope with the trauma she was experiencing from the limitations the stroke placed on her, she began training her brain.

When the stroke victim's wheelchair was wheeled into the training facility on the morning of her first visit, her speech was slurred and her face drooped. Later in the day, when her daughter arrived to take her mother home, she noticed that her mother's speech was clearer and her face didn't droop as much.

Each day, the trainer invited the stroke victim to see herself walking and moving her left arm. At first, this woman couldn't even visualize this scenario. Then two days after she completed her first full course of training, she had a dream in which she saw herself walking. A few weeks later, this client took her first unassisted steps while undergoing physical therapy.

We have already noted that brain training was never intended to be a panacea. It doesn't replace the work of physical therapists, psychotherapists, life coaches, or pastoral counselors, let alone the medical profession. Neither is training your brain a replacement for self-improvement practices such as meditation, tai chi, or yoga. Rather, training balances the brain in a way that enhances the success of these practices, which enables us to fully experience and utilize the information we receive from both our inner and our outer worlds.

Sometimes brain training may not bring about a direct improvement in someone's condition, yet balancing the brain provides a basis on which a variety of different healing and self-help modalities are finally able to function effectively. Doctors, psychiatrists, therapists, counselors involved in drug and alcohol rehabilitation, practitioners of alternative medicine, and many other professionals find their work with patients who have a balanced brain is more effective.

Training our brain helps us surpass ourselves in our endeavor to grow personally. Take someone who meditates regularly in order to improve their functioning. Such a person may not have a balanced brain, but the meditation helps them learn control. As a result of increased control over their thoughts and emotions, they may enjoy a considerable degree of happiness and contentment. If their neural network is then balanced, they are able to derive much more from their meditation. Brain training facilitates a much greater awareness, allowing them to journey further toward fulfillment because they don't have to use so much of their energy to overcome their imbalance.

In other words, for some people brain training functions like a pitchfork in the hands of a gardener, pulling up the sod and loosening the ground in preparation for whatever crops are to be planted. The training prepares the mental and emotional ground. Then the other professions do the sowing, watering, weeding, pruning, and ultimately harvesting.

21

A Journey into Consciousness

TO TAKE RESPONSIBILITY FOR THE QUALITY of our life requires an increase in our awareness of what's going on in our inner world and how we either react negatively to or respond constructively to the world around us. We can only take responsibility for our life to the degree we are really aware of the ins and outs of our circumstances and how we interact with them.

There's much talk these days about increasing the level of consciousness on the planet. It's a nice thing to work toward, but it's difficult to accomplish because we can't increase our consciousness if our neural network is stuck in patterns that won't allow for such an increase. When we are stuck, we are stuck. We don't move much in consciousness or otherwise.

The brain includes a layer between the unconscious and the conscious that is a patterning, a network. It's this network that brain training can affect, so that we utilize optimal patterns rather than unhelpful patterns. For this reason, a balanced brain is an effective starting point to increase consciousness. Getting the network working well is the foundation on which a more conscious world can be built.

People invest a lot of time, money, and effort trying to become more consciousness by reading books, listening to lectures, and attending retreats. Despite all of this effort, unless a person is able to establish fundamentally new brain patterns, no sooner do they determine to make a change than they find themselves repeating the same old behavior. A person may feel calm and collected throughout an entire weeklong retreat, yet not be in the front door of their home more than five minutes before they revert to the unconscious behavior patterns that dominated before they attended the retreat.

Automatic functioning is difficult to overcome, though not impossible. With a great deal of determination, it's possible to modify the effect of some brain patterns, but often this is simply a shifting of energy. The change is cosmetic. For instance, a client remarked, "My dad never drank again after his heart attack. They told him that if he drank, it would kill him. But sometimes I wished he would have, because sometimes he was almost better when he was drunk than when he was sober." The change this father had accomplished was only surface deep. His demanding demeanor hadn't changed. In Alcoholics Anonymous, they call such a person a "dry drunk." The expression points to the essence of the issue, which is a brain energy imbalance.

All of us want to be more conscious because, when we are in a conscious frame of mind, we feel better and we have more power in whatever circumstances we find ourselves. If we are contented, we're more likely to handle stress well. We're more likely to be thoughtful, more likely to be compassionate—and more likely to reap the side benefits of good health and longevity.

If you visit a guru, a pastor, or a therapist who doesn't look healthy, there's a high probability this person has a brain imbalance. When they are preaching, they are really preaching to their own imbalance. Consider the fact such individuals often devote their life to the business of personal transformation. If, after years of working on themselves, these specialists still aren't really seeing the benefits they ought to be seeing, what chance is there for the average person? This is where brain training has a huge advantage over other modalities— as we have seen, not necessarily as a replacement for those modalities, but as a means of kick-starting the transformation process.

Harnessing the Transformative Power of Meditation

Many studies have examined the effects of meditation on people who are depressed, anxious, unable to sleep, in pain, or suffering from a pathology such as cancer. It's clear from these studies that meditation can help a variety of conditions.

Meditation has also long been recognized as an effective tool for personal growth. By focusing on our breathing, trying to be conscious, working with consciousness groups, and seeking to witness and understand our behavior in everyday situations, we encourage the brain to develop more-satisfying patterns.

Still, the process of transformation through meditation is slow and can take years, even decades. In this era when we are accustomed to a quick fix, how many of us are likely to follow through long enough to see lasting results? The reality is that few of us in western society are able to meditate effectively enough to have a significant impact on our condition. This is where brain training can help. It's not a quick fix, but it helps us to move into a state of balance that will enable meditation to be more effective for us.

Meditation is a mode of being, rather than something we do. To be successful, the meditative process requires us to allow ourselves to be held by the universe. To be held is to be in a place where we don't cling to anything for safety and where our fear isn't dominant. However, it's not the kind of state people generally have in mind when they speak of "surrender." When most talk about surrender, it's something they do that requires effort, instead of effortlessly letting go.

This is different from allowing ourselves simply to be held by the universe—allowing ourselves to *be*. When we allow ourselves to be held and to be, it provides us with all the safety and comfort we need. We are in a place where we can receive, without any need for manipulation or any attempt to control situations.

It's not easy for people who are attached to security and control to simply rest in the arms of the universe. Most of us in western society can't do it. We think that to *be* requires some kind of effort, some formula we have to follow. We are so accustomed to *doing* that just *being* is like asking us to walk on the moon when we have never even been to the moon.

Brain training can help at this point. To *be* is much easier for us when our neural network is balanced. When the brain is out of balance, we are constantly trying to "get somewhere" or to somehow "fix" things. Once we are in a state of homeostasis, striving to be somewhere other than where we are ceases.

To be in a state of *being* is to be wide open to receive. Being open to receive is to reach out from a point of essence. It's the difference between living our life from a love of life, or living our life in fear. *Being* is a state that's both powerful and extremely resilient, like shoe leather is strong and tough simply by virtue of being shoe leather. We don't have to try to be powerful, tough, or resilient. It's the natural result of being in homeostasis.

In such a state, we pick up on information we need in order to live fulfilled lives. Whatever guidance we may require and whatever pathology we may be experiencing, the information we need usually simply comes to us, and comes virtually effortlessly. We receive it much like we received our life when we entered the world, coming to us as a gift without our having to do anything to construct it ourselves. Living in this manner, if something is needed in our life, we are shown what's needed. We are led into just the situations we require, but it's all quite effortless. There's no struggle, no agonizing. Indeed, if we are open to it, the whole of life teaches us how to become our deeper, more conscious self, though we will only grasp its lessons to the degree our brain is balanced.

Even when a person's brain state is constantly changing and they only receive glimpses of the pure state of heaven, a glimpse of something so peaceful and so wonderful is all that's needed to evoke a basic contentment and hope. When we embrace this state of contentment, it helps the change we seek in our life to happen. Even if it doesn't appear to be happening, we can trust that we are right where we are intended to be.

Often in brain training, when the brain first sees itself, an area of our life we might really want to change doesn't at first change. Instead, change happens in other places. Only later does the specific area we hoped to change respond. Sometimes a particular area of our life we want to change can only be accessed via a circuitous route. This has to do with how the neural patterns originally formed, coupled with the multiple layers that may have been added since the original imbalance occurred. If more than brain training is required to facilitate our transformation into the glory of our full potential, then we will be guided to exactly what will help us. It will happen naturally, effortlessly, in the right timing.

Understanding Effortlessness

If you are a parent and you pick your baby up from its crib and hold it in front of you, it's likely to squirm, attempting to get right up against you. The baby isn't passive. It expects the parent is going to be there to provide what it needs. The baby isn't trying to make you love it; there is just a natural trust that you will.

When we feel loved—when we have no doubt we are loved—everything we do flows from love. For instance, suppose we have a decision to make. What if we were to make our decision out of love instead of fear? What would the decision look like? Well, it would come from a peaceful place. We would have a sense of being guided, so that we don't have to agonize about the choice we are making but can trust it to be the best we are capable of at the time.

When love fills our heart, the world opens up before us. We realize there are countless possibilities, and we become open to whichever of them the universe deems fitting. We are genuinely open to whatever life sends our way, and our "whatever" has no restrictions.

Even if someone comes into our life who seems to be an obstacle in our path, we welcome them. Instead of resisting them or fearing them, we see them through the eyes of love. This enables us to embrace them exactly where they are on their journey, without trying to change them or cause them to be elsewhere.

This is what it means to be conscious. We accept others, and we connect with them right where they are, no matter how unconscious their state. If they seem like a significant irritant, we regard them as an educator. We take heed because they may be mirroring something to us that we can learn from. Sometimes that "something" is simply gratitude that we are no longer living unconsciously like them—a gratitude that's free of any sense of superiority.

22

Healthy Intimacy

"THIS MORNING MY HUSBAND TALKED TO ME more meaningfully than he ever has in all our years together," a wife reported after her husband began training his brain.

Daryl didn't care to dance, and when his wife Sarah, who enjoyed dancing, tried to drag him onto the dance floor, he always resisted and at best would dance only one dance. You can imagine how surprised Sarah was when the weekend after Daryl started brain training, while listening to music as they were fixing dinner, he grabbed her hand and said, "Let's dance."

Sarah began noticing other changes in the way Daryl related to her. She longed for him to dress nicely, but he had never been particular about the clothes he wore. As brain training progressed, even how he dressed changed. Now, he wanted to look his best and respected Sarah's understanding of what this meant in terms of dress. The many comments he received from friends and coworkers affirmed to him he was on the right path. His life had changed.

Once the initial chemistry between two people has worked its magic, how do they prevent their relationship from becoming routine? How can they keep the romance and passion alive?

To keep a relationship vibrantly alive requires that we become *aware*—conscious of the patterns of behavior into which we so easily slip, attuned to how our words and actions affect our partner, and alert to what matters to this person we claim to love. In this way, we show deep respect for the other, and we are ever mindful of the importance of this respect. As a consequence, both within our own being and in the way we relate as a couple, we are alive and fully present.

Brain training injected new life into Sarah and Daryl's twenty-two year marriage. The difference lay in the fact Daryl was becoming alive within himself, aware of his partner's desires, more grateful for how she enhanced his life, and therefore attentive.

How We Fail to Connect

As the years go by, couples often find their passion for each other wanes. Physical expression of their love in many cases becomes less frequent, and sometimes they go for periods of time without sex.

Most of the decline in sexual interest between a couple has little to do with their physical ability to enjoy sex. It has to do with what's going on in their head. The primary instrument of our sexuality is the *brain*.

One of the reasons sex often diminishes in relationships is that sexual functioning in everyday life is much more complex than simply experiencing desire for each other on a date. Healthy sexual functioning is directly linked to the wider context of how we relate to each other in everyday situations and the respect we hold for each other. If the context isn't emotionally pleasing, we are turned off by the *thought* of sex. It's what's happening in our brain that's paramount.

Consider a situation in which you move to a new house and order an expensive piece of furniture that's scheduled to be delivered cash-on-delivery in a few days. When you open your mail that evening, you realize you forgot about the car insurance because the bill went to your old address and the payment is due tomorrow. You don't have the money in the bank to pay for the furniture as well as the insurance, so you have to cancel the furniture, which happens to be a piece your mate particularly wanted. Although you are in a loving relationship and everything is going great between you, how likely do you suppose your mate is to be passionately intimate with you when you explain the need to cancel the delivery? Depending on the manner in which this happens, there may be intimacy, but it's likely to be less passionate. Stressful situations generally don't promote libido.

Or take a man who is presented with a crisis in his career. He has a stunningly beautiful wife whom he adores, and they are both looking forward to a romantic evening. But at work that day, he learns he is being laid off. In a tight job market and with little in the bank to cushion him, not to mention a large mortgage and car payments, how passionate is he likely to be that evening? No matter how beautiful a woman is, and no matter how much he appreciates his mate, the crisis he now faces will likely short-circuit his libido. The stress of the situation—the sheer weight on his *mind*—eclipses robust physical and emotional connection.

The stress of our modern society, particularly in a time of economic recession, tends to make people increasingly uptight, which has a tightening effect on the muscles. The tighter we become, the less sexual expression we seem to seek. Men and women who lose their sex drive usually find that it revives if they balance and harmonize their brain. The homeostasis of a balanced brain decreases anxiety, making it easier for them to enter into deep relaxation. Anxiety is a killer of libido, whereas relaxation encourages the free flowing of desire, along with blood flow, and thus the ability to perform.

It's not just the trials of everyday existence that can torpedo sexual desire. Simply not behaving in caring ways toward each other affects sexual desire also. For instance, when Daryl repeatedly refused to venture onto the dance floor at an event that afforded an opportunity to do something his wife thoroughly enjoyed, how do you suppose this affected her desire for him sexually? When Sarah longed to share her thoughts and feelings at the end of the day, but her husband didn't talk to her, do you imagine it made her feel more amorous toward him or less?

When a couple come together, they either increasingly work to tune each other in, or they gradually tune each other out. They tune their partner in or tune them out according to their ability to tune into themselves and be honest and real with themselves. Self-respect enables respect for another.

Balancing the brain is a crucial aspect of being able to tune into ourselves and therefore into a partner. If our brain is out of balance, we simply won't be aware of how we are relating. One of the greatest problems in relationships is that people are oblivious of their own behavior and the cues given them by their mate.

Daryl is a classic example of how lack of self-awareness results in an inability to be intimate with a mate. He had been tuning his wife out for years, then wondered why she was rarely interested in making love with him. When he began tuning her in and saw the value in her and in their connection with each other, the relationship shifted into a higher gear.

The reality is, Daryl didn't know how to tune his wife in because the imbalance in his brain put a cap on his awareness. Without awareness of himself, he was incapable of being aware of his wife's desires—incapable of intimacy.

Balance and harmony are the very essence of sexuality and sexual expression. The greater the balance and harmony in a person's brain, the greater their ability to "know" themselves and to identify what they really want in a shared life. The greater the self-awareness, the deeper the emotional intimacy, and the more complete the gratification of sexual expression.

Training for Intimacy

Anxiety is a nervous kind of alertness that's driven by fear, so that we are always on guard. There's another form of alertness, which we might call presence, that's confident, caring, and keenly aware of a partner's real value.

Brain training can help couples open up to each other because it lessens the anxiety people feel about themselves in each other's presence. Anxiety not only blocks much of our creativity, it blocks our ability to really be present with someone.

Daryl had a high level of anxiety. In fact, it was his anxiety that gave him his tremendous drive in the business world. But this same anxiety was also his Achilles' heel when it came to how he related to his wife Sarah.

As a result of brain training, there was a wonderful spinoff from Daryl's reduced anxiety. With his anxiety gone, he found his level of awareness increasing. This enabled him to explore a more vital connection with his wife. Because he was becoming more conscious, he was paying attention to Sarah's true human value as if she were actually a real person like himself and not simply his sidekick.

The Differences Between the Sexes Are Real

Males and females approach sex differently because their brains are different in some fundamental ways. The differences require considerable adjustment before couples learn to enjoy each other free of anxiety. In fact, we are quite different in a variety of ways, though these differences are expressed on a continuum, so that what may be true of a particular man or woman may not be so true of another.

Since a majority of males and females tend to be at opposite poles of the continuum, it's possible to generalize, as long as we are aware that individuals of both sexes can be found at all points in between these poles. While recognizing that people are at different places on the continuum, it's generally the case that a female seeks to become emotionally involved with a male before she enters into a sexual relationship. A male, on the other hand, wants to get into a physical relationship and then see if he wants to become emotionally involved.

The reason for the differences between male and female is that our brains work differently. For one thing, the female corpus callosum, which is the central band of nerves connecting the left and right hemispheres of the brain, is more permeable. This enables females to switch easily from context to detail. Because of this ability to go back and forth between the big picture and the details, a female needs the requirements of both sides of her brain satisfied before she can become truly passionate.

Of prime importance to a female is security, both physical and emotional. Her brain is wired this way because for generations she had to go to the waterhole with her offspring and make sure they weren't attacked by dangerous animals and hostile individuals. She required a permeable corpus callosum to allow her to go back and forth between the task at hand and awareness of her children and any threat from the environment. She could easily go from detail to context and back.

The male, since his corpus callosum is less permeable, is more likely to focus on one particular aspect of the relationship. He tends to "lock down" on the physical side, leaving the emotional side of his brain out of the picture in initial encounters. Males are driven more by their occipital lobes, which are thirty percent larger than those of a female. The male's occipital lobes, which control vision, have driven him from prehistoric times when he hunted. To this day, he wants to see something that excites him.

We often put each other down, with the woman putting the man down for "only wanting one thing," and the man putting the woman down for "always needing to talk about everything." But there's nothing wrong with the differences between the sexes. In fact, rather than being a cause for an impasse, the differences can serve as a tool for increasing intimacy, and hence passion, once couples are willing to allow these differences to change them.

Although males and females seem to want different things, the fact is they want the same things. While it's true that with a man it's often very much about sex, and with a woman it's more likely to be about emotional security, the reality is that both are fulfilled only when there is both passionate sex and emotional connection. The differences between the sexes, when honored instead of compromised, are precisely what can drive us both to develop into whole human beings who are capable of profound connection interlaced with romance and passion. We just come at it from different approaches.

Though we associate sexual desire more with males, when a woman feels secure and her life is in balance, her sex drive tends to increase. In fact, once the female's desire for security is satisfied, the male often finds he has less sex drive than his partner. And sometimes the male has more need for ongoing security than does the female, as many men find when their wife or girlfriend leaves them unexpectedly and functions perfectly well without them.

Two people decide they are interested in each other. If the male wants to engage in sexual activity and the female wants to be sure of what his commitment is, what should they do? Instead of expecting to enter into a sexual relationship, what if the two were to embark on an open discussion about how they feel about sex and really explain to each other the kind of sexual expression they enjoy, with nothing held back. This is the approach a person with a balanced brain may take. In other words, there would be total frankness in a completely judgment-free atmosphere where no one is allowed to say, "You need *what?*"

When the brain is out of balance, it can't afford to be aware. To be aware requires energy, but this energy is being used to sustain itself in an out-of-balance condition. The situation is unbearable if the person has no solution, and so the brain may prefer a numbed state.

Relationships challenge us to grow and become people who are more balanced in every aspect of our life—people who use more of our brain, harnessed by the mind, to achieve increasing wisdom in how we relate to each other.

23

When Sex Becomes a Crime

IF AN IMBALANCE IN THE BRAIN can result in a lack of libido, a different pattern of imbalance can also generate a desperate need for sex in both males and females. When this occurs, people attempt to use sex as a way to offset the imbalance they are experiencing.

When stress causes an imbalance in the brain to the point that it affects sexual functioning, it not only diminishes our functioning, it can also make sexual expression less healthy and fulfilling. This happens because, even as we find ourselves becoming less sexual toward our partner, we discover we still have a great need to be a sexual being. To deny our sexuality is like trying to put a tight lid on something that's generating pressure. This can cause our sexuality to come out in ways we are ashamed of. For example, sexual desire that isn't acknowledged tends to manifest in compulsive activity such as pornography, prostitution, and 900 number erotic phone calls. Shame arises because people for the most part don't want to be seen using pornography or visiting a prostitute. It's all undercover. Anytime anything is permitted only in the dark, you have to ask how healthy it is.

Feeling *driven* to have sex, almost compulsively, is often the result of a sympathetic dominance, where the person is in a fight-or-flight mode and lacks the ability to make executive decisions that take into consideration all the factors involved in a situation. In such a situation, the act of sex creates a feeling of safety by producing a temporary sensation of balance. But the respite achieved is short-lived.

Brain training helps sexual dysfunction and can have a life-changing impact on sexual deviance. Brain training is effective with the sex offender because he isn't the evil animal society has been led to believe. He's a person who is using sex as a drug. Because he has grown up with his foot on the brake all his life, the only way he can make the car go is to slam down the gas pedal. It's the same for people who feel a need to visit a prostitute even when they are in a relationship. A sex offence usually doesn't originate with a lack of willpower, being immoral, or disrespect for women. These are all symptoms. The cause invariably lies in a heavy imbalance, for which individuals attempt to compensate.

Society considers a sex offender to have an incurable condition. But the sex offender isn't fundamentally different from the person who uses drugs. Why would somebody start using drugs? They use drugs as a way to artificially bring the brain into balance. People zone out on television for the same reason. They don't have to think about anything as long as they can sit zombie-like in front of the television. One person goes out and shops in order to cope with the imbalance in their brain, while another turns to gambling. All these behaviors are attempts to increase the activity in the area of the brain that's underactive, in order to compensate for excess activity in other areas.

Addiction to sex works in a similar way. For some, the attempt to use sex as a means of artificially bringing their brain into balance takes the form of having a variety of partners, to the point that sleeping with different people becomes an addiction. Others can only step on the gas pedal if there is a forceful element to the sexual act, which is the case of the person who is likely to become a sex offender. Whatever the particular form the addiction takes, it's a way to bring the brain into a temporary state of balance, thus relieving the individual's distress for a while.

Brain trainers have evidence of shopaholics and gamblers being changed, and also of sex offenders being changed. People who were spending all their money calling 900 numbers and getting into serious debt have been able to end their addiction. Teens and individuals in their twenties who couldn't focus on their studies because they couldn't curb watching pornography on the internet have also been able to change.

In the case of pedophiles, there are not yet long-term studies, though we await these with interest. A state corrections institution will likely be the place we will see such a study in the future. It's only a matter of time until an official has enough courage to move forward to help people with this brain imbalance. Simultaneously, such an official will be protecting society.

Making Sense of Pedophilia

The drive to sexually abuse another person is a difficult pattern for therapy to remove. But the pattern is clearly evident in a brain assessment, and it can be addressed successfully with training that balances and brings harmony to the patterns of the entire brain. However, sexual abuse is a bigger issue for the victim, where there are many levels of post-traumatic stress. For this reason, sexual offences as they relate to the victim will be treated in a separate chapter.

Unlike sexual dysfunction, sexual deviance is considered by society to be all but incurable. For instance, pedophiles are labeled for life. As far as society is concerned, it's what they *are*.

I can certainly understand this attitude. When I worked at a mental health institute in a pastoral counseling clinical training experience years ago, the one type of counselee I couldn't deal with was a pedophile. I felt such harsh judgment toward them, as if they were the epitome of evil. Offering a compassionate ear was impossible for me. How could someone want to abuse a child? I thought about my own children. The idea that someone could use them sexually enraged me.

As part of the clinical counseling training experience, I explained how difficult it was for me to work with pedophiles. I couldn't imagine such a thing. Not only could I not relate to someone abusing a child, I couldn't imagine myself being with a female young enough to be my daughter.

It was only when I started looking at brain patterns years later that I realized a person doesn't become a pedophile because they lack values, but because they have a brain imbalance. When I saw with my own eyes the tormented state of a pedophile's brain, and realized this state had likely been inflicted on them in their own childhood, I was brought to my knees in terms of shame for the way I had condemned such individuals. Condemnation isn't helpful, whereas understanding is.

Protecting children is absolutely essential. Judgment of the pedophile as incurable and less than human is an entirely different matter. I had to face the fact I was so judgmental because my own neural activity was high in exactly the opposite areas of the brain. Even as the pedophile's neural activity is low in certain neighborhoods of the brain, mine was high in those same neighborhoods. This is why some of us are so much more judgmental than others. Whether we are considering a pedophile or the person who argues such a person should be executed, the only difference between the two is that their brain has an equal imbalance in the opposite direction.

Realizing that pedophilia and harsh condemnation of the pedophile are two sides of the same coin clears up a common misunderstanding bequeathed to us from a flawed view of the human psyche. We often hear that when an individual is vehemently opposed to certain kinds of people, it's because they have suppressed a tendency in themselves to exhibit the same behavior. For instance, those who gay bash are considered to be homophobic because they are suppressing a desire to experience homosexuality themselves. It is sometimes true that we attack most what we suppress in ourselves. There are countless examples of public figures who have loudly condemned sexual impropriety, only to be caught engaging in identical activity. But suppression of our own tendencies is by no means the *only* reason people rage at pedophilia, homosexuality, or sexual license. To hate pedophiles and sexual libertines can simply mean that *we have the opposite imbalance.*

A pedophile commits an act of pedophilia because their imbalance drives them to try to balance their brain by "stepping on the gas," which takes the form of seeking control. This is a condition that brain training can address. It's terribly important our society comes to understand that both sexual deviance and harsh judgment of the deviant is about brain imbalance and disharmony. If we once become aware of this, it will change how we respond to people who exhibit such an imbalance.

Because what a pedophile does is against the law, the person can be arrested for their imbalance. But a person whose imbalance causes them to want to see pedophiles executed is, by legal standards, doing nothing wrong unless they act on their intolerance. Of course, the reason many don't take action is that their brain screams at them, "You'll be in the same correctional institute as the pedophile!" But according to the teaching of Jesus, to wish another dead because we so hate them is just as bad as murdering them in terms of any true understanding of higher consciousness. Wanting to kill someone is on the same unconscious level as the act we believe causes the individual to deserve being killed. In other words, both individuals are in the grip of the same kind of self-destructive pattern, just on the other side of the fence.

We have to get away from the idea that people do bad things because they are thoroughly evil. Let me illustrate why this is important by citing the case of somebody who suffers from post-traumatic stress disorder and flies into a rage easily. Afterwards, the person invariably feels an immense amount of shame. Why? Didn't they understand that if they went into a rage, they were going to do the wrong thing? Yes, they understood. They knew that if they unleashed their anger, it wouldn't have a good outcome. It's their understanding—their sense of values—that made them feel terrible later. We wouldn't want to execute such a person because we realize that the problem isn't a lack of understanding or values, but an imbalance. Well, it's no different with sexual deviance. Help is what's needed, not hatred.

Date Rape

Part of the reason for widespread sexual deviance is that cultural values haven't caught up with the fact we are sexual beings seeking respectful ways to exercise our sexuality. As a society, we want to participate in sex, but we don't want to engage in a thorough discussion about it publicly yet. Because we won't discuss most forms of sexual deviance openly, such behavior stays mostly underground.

However, date rape is one of the areas in which, at last, there is growing public awareness of the dangers. Because of increased open discussion of the topic, young women are realizing that date rape isn't just a "one off," where the man became too sexually stimulated and lost control. The same male may date rape many women, all the while claiming it was the woman's fault for leading him to a state of overstimulation.

Because men are sprinters, it's true they are easily stimulated, and in our current culture there's no lack of stimulation. It screams at us from billboards, the pages of magazines, the lives of celebrities, television, and the more suggestive way of dressing that's popular today. In years past, women didn't explore all the ways they could enhance their sexuality, such as facelifts, breast implants, buttocks uplifts, and tummy tucks. Now such enhancements are commonplace. All of this appeals to men, who are visually stimulated far more than women because, as we have already mentioned, the occipital lobes are thirty percent larger in the male.

The stimulation males are subjected to isn't the *reason* they take advantage of women—though, in order to alleviate their guilt, men will argue it is. Were we to assess the brain of a perpetrator of date rape, his frontal lobes would reveal a severe lack of ability to self-stimulate. There's also a high likelihood he has an attention deficit problem. In other words, no matter the nature of sexual deviance, it tends to originate in an imbalance of the neural network. This reality makes date rape all the more unacceptable because now that we know the source of this behavior is likely a brain imbalance, such an imbalance should be investigated and then addressed.

Men with a balanced brain, in which all the neighborhoods are in harmony, don't tend to exploit the power differential between themselves and females. They don't misuse their physical strength, and they don't manipulate a woman for self-gratification. But men with an imbalance may manipulate a woman, using any means to gratify themselves without regard for her. They recognize she wants to know there's emotional connection, and so they give the impression they are emotionally available for the one purpose of achieving sexual consummation. Such a man takes what he wants, then disappears, because he can get away with it as long as the woman doesn't recognize her vulnerability to manipulation.

A balanced and harmonized brain enables a man to see a woman to whom he is attracted through the lens of love rather than as an object to manipulate. A brain in homeostasis causes a person to see others from a vantage that respects our interdependence and interconnectedness.

When a man recognizes his interconnectedness, he treats a date not as prey but as a precious individual who is to be honored and respected. If a woman wishes to delay physical intimacy, a man with a balanced brain doesn't try to manipulate her. Neither does he interpret her postponement of sex in a negative way. At the same time, a woman with a balanced brain doesn't suppress her own passion and withhold. The balance and harmony of both the male and the female brain is then reflected in the balance of power in the relationship, so that the couple's interaction is mutual, respectful of the limits of the other, and healthy.

Sexual deviance often revolves around a *lack of power*. The appropriate use of power flows naturally when the brain is in balance, with all parts of the neural system functioning harmoniously. When a person uses sex to overpower another person, it's a very different experience of sexuality than intimacy shared in mutuality. It isn't sex, actually; it's assault. Such an inappropriate use of power is almost always a misguided attempt to correct a brain imbalance by means of a short-lived thrill achieved through control over another human being.

The Different Strengths of Male and Female Brains

One of the reasons sexual devience is only now coming to light as a scourge of society is that for generations it's been possible to hide such deviance under the cloak of patriarchy and the assumed right of males to dominate females. This is at last changing in many societies and is set to crumble on a global scale as the world becomes increasingly interconnected.

Today, more women are in positions of leadership in the world than ever in history. This is a good thing for the future of the planet because women have certain skills suited to leadership that men are short on.

The fact that women haven't tended to dominate throughout much of history says nothing about their ability to lead. It has much more to do with cultural roles traditionally assigned to them because of the necessity of bearing children, coupled with the fact that males by virtue of their sheer size and strength are more suited to the hunt and the defense of the tribe.

The male brain is a great analytical tool, but a female brain is often more capable of moving back and forth between detail and context. When it comes to leadership, difficult as it may be for males to accept, a woman whose brain is balanced and in harmony may be better equipped. This is because leadership is best accomplished when both the left and right hemispheres of the brain are fully engaged, so that the individual can switch which hemisphere they are using in a flash, according to the particular task at hand. Women have better perspective when it comes to leadership because a female brain can go from functioning primarily on the left to functioning on the right, then back again, much faster than a male brain.

We noted earlier that the source of the flexibility of the female brain is the corpus callosum. As the infant grows in the mother, testosterone is absorbed through the corpus callosum and can impair its permeability. Consequently, the female corpus callosum is more permeable than that of a male, which facilitates shifting between the left and right hemispheres of the brain. This enables the female brain to more easily put things in context. Males become focused on the details, more easily losing sight of the larger picture, which is why we often hear it said that men think in boxes. When men think about cars, their mind is on cars. When they think about football, they are focused on football. And when it's hunting season, they are preoccupied with hunting. Females, on the other hand, readily switch back and forth from the wider context to details.

We also noted that a feature of the male brain is that it tends to become "locked down" more easily. This is why seventy-five percent of autistic children are male.[24] In autistic individuals, the corpus callosum isn't permeable, which means the individual can't move energy from one side of the brain to the other.[25] If you can't think from one side of your brain to the other, you may be exceptional in math, but you might not understand a joke because it requires switching quickly to the other side of the brain. You have a hyper ability to focus on detail, but your ability to see things in context is severely restricted. I hypothesize this is a contributing factor in autism.

If autism tends to develop in the male because the male brain can lock down more readily, in the female bipolar tends to develop more readily because the corpus callosum becomes too permeable and goes back and forth too readily. A woman may be really happy, but then she becomes really sad. This tendency is worsened by the difference in the underlying hormonal factories in the male and female, which in the female support going back and forth too quickly. If a man encounters this problem, it usually comes at a later stage of life, when it can be more severe.

Women take greater responsibility for their bodies, going for regular gynecological and breast examinations. Men don't like to talk about prostate problems because they are locked down on one side of the brain and don't see their health in context. It's a macho thing that stems from our hunting and gathering days. If a man was in pain, he didn't get up and hunt that day. If a woman was in pain, she was much more likely to get up because, if she didn't, the family went hungry and the children untended. The problem is exacerbated today by the fact we don't have to go far to hunt down a fast food restaurant. In our technological society when we don't have to hunt, we need to evolve healthy filters and flexibility so we can accept input culturally and use it wisely. Brain training helps people develop appropriate filters and flexibility.

24

Your Past Is Not Your Present

NO MATTER WHAT MAY HAVE BEFALLEN US in the past, brain training is designed to free us from patterns in our neural network that tether us to the pain we have endured.

We are not the sum of our past painful experiences.

Beneath any agony we may have experienced, there is a healthy person who emerges once our brain is restored to a state of balance and harmony.

A woman in her early sixties whose name is Marjorie had only a fragment of a memory of being sexually abused as a young child. Studies have shown that the power of suggestion when a person is relaxed is huge. For instance, in one study children were induced into a relaxed state then told stories, which they were asked to remember. For years afterwards, the children honestly thought they had lived this memory. They could smell things, see the colors, and describe the setting as if they had been present, yet it never happened. Just because someone says they have a memory doesn't mean it's accurate. Sometimes it isn't easy to determine whether a trauma such as incest really happened. A brain assessment helps to clarify the potential for incest.

Marjorie's brain assessment revealed she had indeed suffered a childhood infringement. Her story of brain training shows how our past cannot limit us if we don't want it to, no matter how devastating this past may have been.

Creating New Pathways

For the past eleven years, Marjorie had found herself in a constant state of hyper-vigilance, which was taking a toll on her body. "I was literally slogging through life, barely putting one foot in front of the other," she recalls. Emotionally and financially, she felt overwhelmed, which caused her to experience constant nausea. Marjorie's initial brain assessment verified the exhaustion she felt.

Marjorie's physical exhaustion helped her release the tension and anxiety connected to always having to be in control and "performing." She was now so exhausted, she simply couldn't perform any longer. Her energy was so low that some days she would wake up at 6:30 AM, but by 9 AM she had to go back to bed. It seemed to her that feeling so drained and depleted was the universe's "way to get me out of the way."

During the process of training her brain, Marjorie tapped into the deep roots of embarrassment that grew from being abused. "I suppose I was six or seven when I first began planting the seeds of embarrassment and by ten they were deeply rooted," she says. "I didn't fully comprehend what happened to me, only that it was embarrassing and made me feel sick. I hung my head in shame."

Over time the roots of embarrassment penetrated so deeply that they skewed Marjorie's ability to discern what should be embarrassing and what's normal. "It sometimes takes me days to dig out and identify the roots of embarrassment that spring up in the most unusual experiences," she explains.

Marjorie is hypersensitive to her trauma history. She is aware that it colors her interaction with others. "I am transferring this emotional memory to other relationships and other feelings," she says. "Someone I trust tells me they will do something, but they don't follow through. I go away embarrassed and ashamed for having an expectation of them. Then the real action starts, as I begin the game of blame, targeting myself. 'I picked the wrong friend. I miscommunicated. I screwed up.' The self-hatred kicks into high gear and I experience nausea. I am physically in pain, and I am emotionally paralyzed."

At a brain training session, the tones of the computer program vibrate in her ears. Calming herself, Marjorie begins to respond to the comforting sounds of release and healing. "I consciously practice compassion," she recounts. "It doesn't matter what I encountered or how I judged myself. What matters is the powerful healing of the sounds and tones."

During the three weeks following her first ten-session brain training intensive, Marjorie finds her brain readjusting. Her mind is much clearer, especially when it comes to identifying the areas of her life in which she wants to experience transformation and growth.

It takes courage to confront the trauma of childhood, especially sexual abuse. Over half of all who experience sexual abuse also suffer extreme symptoms of post-traumatic stress disorder. Brain training is a safe way to meet this challenge and create new pathways not based on old pain. As Marjorie explains, "I am safe and protected in this process—surrounded by beloved friends, family, and the brain trainers."

A Cleansing Process

Marjorie's brain had adopted a pattern that enabled her to survive at the time she was being abused. But her frozen mode, which kept her from feeling the immensity of the injustice that was perpetrated against her, later in life prevented her from embracing life with her whole being. "Today I am increasingly aware of the extent to which, over the years, I held myself back from moving forward because of my fears and my abuse," she says. "Because of brain training I am shifting that behavior. I am actively seeking all the richness of life. I am asking to receive and grateful when it manifests. I am peaceful and safe receiving. This is a remarkable behavior change."

Marjorie sees brain training as similar to being handed a gift in wrapping paper. "I could have chosen to ignore it and leave the wrapping intact," she says. "I could have half-heartedly gone to a few sessions, and then quietly never gone back. Instead, I chose to open the gift. I wanted to transform. No cost—time, money, or energy— was too great. I was ready."

The process unfolds like an undulating ocean, a current of continual healing. Even when you are not in a brain training session, the memory of the protocol tones lingers and reverberates through your awakening cells. At the end of the process is the gold of alchemical transformation.

You see who you have already become and what you might yet become. You see yourself a year from now, five years from now, encountering yourself as someone whose life has dramatically shifted. You meet yourself in a future of possibilities.

Rediscovering Our Innocence

The power of brain training is that as balance and harmony are restored to the brain, we rediscover our essential being and realize it is completely intact despite all that has befallen us.

Marjorie is now able to see herself in a manner that's uncontaminated by the sexual abuse she experienced. She says, "For most of my life I was blind to who I am. Brain training is allowing me to reclaim my identity and my power."

Only as we mature and gain wisdom do we realize we have the power to set boundaries to our availability. As Marjorie grows in awareness of the effects of trauma, she gains strength to set emotional and relationship boundaries. "Through Al-anon, for many years I practiced setting boundaries," she recalls. "It was effective to a certain extent. With brain training, setting boundaries is easier."

A saying pops into Marjorie's mind: "If it has a big back, it has a big front." This is meaningful to her. "As I face my memories, I peer into the dark foundations of who I am. It is harrowing and yet common human behavior. As I pull the veil from the dark foundations, I simultaneously reveal the brilliant light that is within me. I visualize myself as having a big backyard with lots of memories and skills. As I gain conscious understanding of the effects of my trauma, I develop a corresponding big front yard full of light and happiness."

A new horizon is coming into view for Marjorie. "As I progress through this phase, I am open to becoming a new being," she says. "I haven't the faintest idea of the beautiful being who will emerge following these training sessions. I relax back in the knowledge of the alchemy that is occurring in my brain and body. I have no idea how I am going to emerge. What body will be birthed? It will be a new body, of that I am certain. A new rewired body through brain training."

Marjorie says of this new phase in her life, "Before beginning brain training, I was so out of balance that I had to freeze to function. For so many years my life was a constant struggle tangled with fear. Now I identify where I belong by how easily it unfolds."

The Power of Allowing the Past to Die

When one of Marjorie's brothers phoned to tell her that her father was dying, it brought forth both sadness and peace. For five years he had been failing with Alzheimer's, so their contact had been quite limited. Recently there had been no recognition that she was his daughter and she had not seen her father for a year.

Marjorie's sister wanted her to see her father one more time before he died. "I explained to her that one last glimpse or kiss or embrace is not what I need. I need to hold my father in peace, love, and light every day he is with us on earth and every day he is living eternally. That is what I need. And that is what I am giving myself."

When the phone call came telling of the passing of Marjorie's father, she found herself experiencing a peaceful release of all the cords that connected them. She wrote in her journal. "We are both free, now that he and I have transitioned to new places—him through death and me through brain training. Now that the doors of life have closed on our history together, I celebrate this closing and am grateful that I consciously participated in the closing. Brain training kept me conscious, as did this journal."

Marjorie's father suffered the silence of dementia in his final years. Prior to the silence, he was an eloquent, educated orator. He could quote poetry and Shakespeare from memory, not to mention the Bible. Yet in the latter years, he was silent just like he had instructed her to be throughout her formative years when she had no real idea what was going on. At the funeral, among all the children and grandchildren, Marjorie remained silent. "I had nothing to say, nothing," she recalls. "I knew him for fifty-six years of my life and I had nothing to say." Her silence represented forgiveness and release, and she found herself able to smile as the respectful memories poured forth from her brother, sister, and children. "The funeral was about their tributes, their memories, not about my trauma or me," she says.

Marjorie tried to picture what the funeral, burial, and mourning would have been like had she not experienced brain training. "All I can imagine is a black void. I see myself lost in the void, unable to process my thoughts and feelings because my denial would have been so overwhelming. Instead, session after session, my black void opened in brain training, where I was safe. In the training chair, the maze of my childhood crystallized into a pathway full of meaning."

Becoming the Puppeteer

After her father's death, Marjorie asked herself, "Am I a puppet or the puppeteer?" She realized she had certainly been a puppet. But now, "Through brain training I am becoming the puppeteer, pulling my own strings—gently."

Pulling her own strings was beginning to make a difference in her life. "I have been out of town, doing a professional presentation," she says. "I was confident, focused, and the presentation went well. I stayed balanced and happy. I noticed while presenting that I was much more relaxed and fluent with my thoughts. I also notice a distinct rise in my creativity and ability to translate my thoughts into the written word. My writing is becoming clearer and effortless. I spend much less time agonizing over one word versus another.

I spend much less time picking apart sentences with my perfectionism. I have brain training to thank for my success."

In her journal Marjorie wrote, "I often heard sages, mystics, gurus, and saints speak of an open, loving heart. Now I understand. The glass of gnosis is no longer dark. Now when I approach a relationship or an event or a feeling, I focus on my heart. Is all well with my heart? Is it open like a thousand-petal lotus? My open heart emits information and energy that my mind can barely fathom. It holds more ammunition than my fear can ever trigger. It holds more wisdom than the chatter of my mind can ever provide. It holds more energy than my physical body can ever demand. All is well."

The pace of change in Marjorie's life picks up. "I am able to canter," she says. When she returns to brain training, she notices how adept she has become with her brainpower, able to shift her brain's energy pattern and focus.

Marjorie had always over-processed her feelings about her relationships and events in her life and the lives of her love ones. "Simply put, I talk too much," she says. "I am an extroverted thinker, so I literally think out loud. I process and process until I feel safe. By so doing, I wear out others and myself. I jeopardize relationships. I over-analyze and process until I destroy that which I might love, if I gave myself a chance to allow it to flourish without processing and analysis. But as a result of training my brain, I quiet my mind. I quiet my voice. I live and let live."

25

The Extensive Reach of Brain Training

ONE OF THE MOST AMAZING FEATURES of brain training is the deep level of damage it can address, well beyond what many popular modalities are able to accomplish.

Millions of people in modern society have been cast aside as if they were worthless. They are people who have committed a crime of some kind, which might be an act of violence toward another person or simply an infringement of society's ever-changing whims of what's socially acceptable and sociably punishable.

No one disputes that those who have committed violent crimes and who continue to be violent while incarcerated are beyond the limits of most help currently used in correctional institutions. This is why brain trainers were invited to work with a group of inmates who were repeatedly being written up for violence at a Nevada state correctional facility. These men unleashed their violence at least monthly and many of them weekly. One had been diagnosed as paranoid schizophrenic, others as antisocial or addicted. Could brain training help such individuals? Might brain training even help such individuals while they continue to live inside a dangerous environment contaminated with large amounts of serious dysfunction and violence?

To demonstrate the efficacy of brain training in a dangerous environment, brain trainers had to enter the correctional facility and establish training rooms in cells inside the infirmary. Some of the inmates being trained were men whose demeanor alone screamed, "Danger!" The trainers nevertheless shared a tiny cell for several hours of brain training with each inmate. Like all of us, each inmate had his own personality. One barely spoke during three weeks. One asked questions incessantly. One reported on his progress and noted changes in his thinking every day. Others talked little at first and a lot by the end of the three-week training period.

The trainers first read the men's brain assessments to decipher the precise form of imbalance each of them was suffering. They also noted their specific symptoms.

At the end of the training, they again took brain assessments. In each case the men's symptoms had decreased by over fifty percent and in some of them as much as seventy-five percent. From this the trainers could predict that these men were less likely to be violent, less likely to even go into a rage, and more able to cognitively process, focus, and understand reason.

When these inmates were in training, the trainers didn't know that not one of them had the ability to read well. In fact, most could hardly read at all. They knew what words were, but they couldn't maintain their focus long enough to put the words together in a way that made sense. None could read a paragraph and report on what they had read.

None of the inmates were able to sleep well when training began. None were able to trust easily. They didn't trust people on the inside of the correctional facility and absolutely didn't trust anybody outside their race-based group identity. In fact, it was dangerous for them to have any communication with an inmate from another race. Were they to do so, they would be seen as a traitor to their race. A single communication would result in a punishment, a second would result in a beating, and a third incident of communicating with another race would likely lead to death. So low was the level of trust these men exhibited that they didn't even trust their own families.

None of the inmates could speak with any kind of fluency. Their words were delivered with jerkiness and their sentences were choppy. Consequently, they knew nothing of the mental enrichment and emotional enjoyment of conversation. The only time they talked at all was to obtain what they needed at any given moment. Similarly, the movement of their bodies manifested no flow whatever. Even when they moved slowly and purposefully, their movements lacked flow. Their hands were shaking and there was tightness in their neck, shoulders, and arms—an indicator they were continually on alert. All of these factors were stifling any kind of meaningful self-expression.

These inmates were limited in their interaction with the world and with each other because their brain was locked into a pattern it had found beneficial for survival at some time in the past. Such a pattern likely saved the person's life, probably when they were a child. We know this because the men all exhibited trauma patterns in their brain assessment, from which the trainers could determine approximately when each particular trauma occurred. All of the trauma patterns indicated they occurred at an early age.

How a Person Becomes Incarcerated

It became apparent that although these men were in a correctional facility, the *real* prison they were experiencing was *inside* them.

In each case, the brain assessment conducted on these men revealed that their brain wasn't only unbalanced, it was massively unbalanced. Usually we find energy differences of around ten percent between the various lobes, though at times this may be up to fifty percent. These men exhibited differences that were ten times what we see in the general population!

It's not difficult to see how a little brain training had such a dramatic impact on these men. If you empty a bottle and allow it to become dry, adding only a single drop of water makes it comparatively very wet. When a brain is as unbalanced as the brains of these inmates, even a small amount of training is like adding a drop of water to a dry bottle. You can't help but do a lot of good quickly. Consequently, all six of the inmates who trained experienced a tremendous difference in their lives even after only a handful of sessions.

There was no guarantee that the changes accomplished in the initial sessions would be sustained, as every day all inmates returned to a dangerous environment. It would likely take considerably more training for the improvements these men were seeing to become enduring, which is why the brain trainers stayed three weeks. However, the men immediately began sleeping well, were able to communicate effectively, and weren't so reactive. Now, when someone put pressure on them, they didn't automatically explode. They could sustain themselves without rage. They were able to think through a situation and deal with it more like a normal person deals with such situations.

Becoming calm allowed the men to concentrate. Because they could focus, they were able to start reading and studying; and for the first time in their life, they found they retained the information.

Once these inmates started to read, they made rapid progress. By the end of three weeks of brain training, all were reading proficiently. Was it that they didn't want to read before? No, they all said they had wanted to read and desired to take in information. They had tried and tried to read, but their brain simply wasn't about to concentrate due to the unbalanced pattern in which it was stuck.

When the trainers returned five months later, each of the men was many times further along than after the initial brain training. For example, all were making A's and B's in school, which is pleasing in the case of any student but especially in the case of individuals who couldn't read before. Reading leveled their educational playing field. As a result of their studies, they were able to sit and discuss interesting topics with the trainers.

The changes that occurred weren't simply a matter of people deciding to "shape up" and make better choices in life. These inmates didn't decide in July, "I'm going to be a good conversationalist by December." They had no such intention, and this wasn't the objective of training their brains. The aim was simply to create balance and harmony in the different neighborhoods of the brain. Yet each of the men were educating themselves by the time the trainers returned. Why? Because for the first time they had the option to learn—something their brain simply couldn't do before—and they found it was fun to read and absorb information. People can't make good choices if they don't have the mental and emotional ability to do so.

Brain training is about giving people options. If my brain only allows me one door through which to escape a situation, I'll readily take it. When multiple doors are available, I'll discern my path based on the value it offers me and others.

One of the inmates in the brain training program was part American Indian, in his early twenties, of medium size, but well built. In the initial visit, even though the trainers saw him every day for three hours, they heard no more than perhaps fifteen sentences from him. Now he sat and conversed intelligently for over an hour, telling of how he had scored an A- in college-level English, together with a B+ in math, and had become a teaching assistant in the correctional facility. His excitement bubbled over as he described how his family says he has changed and how pleased he is with these improvements in the quality of his life.

A trainer sits in front of a huge, powerful man who has been diagnosed as a paranoid schizophrenic. The man now talks of the importance of 19th century history and how what happened at that time affected what's unfolding in our century now.

It's amazing to look an inmate in the face and see the difference training a brain can make. When the training first began, to be around this man was frightening because he was so physically powerful and emotionally volatile, yet the trainer wouldn't hesitate to have such a man as his neighbor today. In fact, it would be a pleasure, because if the trainer ever needed to lift something heavy, this would be the person to call for help—not only because of his strength, but also because of his helpful attitude!

Creating Community

The six men who were brain trained were living in a correctional institution in which they had to be constantly on alert or they could be seriously injured and even murdered. They had to protect their belongings at all times and they had to show no weakness, which would be an indication of vulnerability. Working with these men inside a medium security correctional institution rather than in a brain training facility revealed that it's possible to train some-body's brain in the dangerous environment of a prison and not have them regress from the daily pressures of such a setting.

It was notable that at the time of the initial brain training, none of these men looked back at the course of their life and expressed a sense of horror, as if they had been incredibly evil. During the entire three weeks of training, they didn't once talk about why they were arrested. But when the trainers returned after five months, all of the men made statements such as, "I'm not going back to that life. I'm not going to do those things ever again." These were inmates who had all been written up for violence directed toward other inmates or prison staff many times in the past, but not one of them had been written up for a violent act in five months.

The most significant aspect of the transformation these men experienced was that they began to experience their value as human beings and could extend this value into their world. They related to their families and friends in a more positive way. They were from three different races, yet they established a friendship. This was unique in the correctional facility. They held meetings at which they talked about their experience of brain training, and they conducted these meetings openly. In other words, they were putting themselves on the line because they now realized their worth and the importance of connecting as a class to learn valuable life information.

It wasn't only the inmates who benefited from brain training. The warden also had to train his brain to prove the process wasn't harmful. You read about his transformation and the impact this had on the inmates in a previous chapter.

Resistance Dies Hard

You would think that with results like these, brain training would be welcomed with open arms by correctional facilities, rehabilitation centers, and other institutions connected with the justice system. Such is not always the case.

When brain training was introduced into the Nevada prison, many were excited by the fact that inmates were becoming more manageable and less dangerous. However, some of the corrections officers thought the prisoners were there to be punished. They surmised: If you commit a crime, shouldn't you have to pay for it?

The purpose of training the brain of inmates isn't so we can turn them all loose in society. It's so that they can become worthwhile human beings in a safer and more humane correctional system even if they are serving a lifelong sentence. When some of the correctional officers couldn't grasp this concept, the warden had to step in and personally facilitate the training process.

We all have a responsibility to treat others in a way that doesn't project onto them the discomfort we feel because of the issues they raise for us. Our responsibility is to own our discomfort, then seek a solution for this discomfort. The fact that someone is incarcerated isn't an indication they are a failure as a human being, but that they most likely have a brain imbalance. It isn't that they are "bad." However, when a person recognizes that they have a problem, they have a responsibility to seek a solution. Society's responsibility is to recognize their human worth and offer them the kind of help brain training affords.

As a result of training their brain, all of the inmates progressed and some were hugely changed. Some will take their place as positive members of society. If you consider that each criminal affects at least thirty-five to forty people in an extremely negative way, and another sixty in a lesser way, it's surely worthwhile to create a positive person who will come in contact with three or four times this number when released and influence them in a beneficial way.

In 1962, I read a book about how new scientific discoveries are adopted. The author explained that the only way new discoveries are embraced is for the reigning generation, which tends to resist change, to die off. Can we move beyond this? As technology moves faster and faster, our ability to resist change will hopefully break down under the barrage of new developments without having to wait for a generation to pass away. Perhaps technology, which has itself caused some cultural problems, can now help society to change itself for the better.

26

A Glimpse of the Future

WRITING IN *THE NEW YORK TIMES*, columnist Janet Rae-Dupree interviewed Michael J. Gelb, a corporate consultant, who is coauthor with Thomas Edison's great-grandniece Sarah Miller Caldicott of the 2007 book *Innovate Like Edison*.

Says Mr. Gelb, speaking of Leonardo da Vinci, "His was a balanced brain in that he used the left and right hemispheres of his cerebral cortex equally and to their fullest, something I've tried to get people from DuPont and Microsoft and Merck to do over the last 30 years."

Mr. Gelb explains, "Corporate executives today tend to be overly linear, logical, analytical. I'm trying to help them use their intuition and artistic capabilities. If you want to compete in the challenging world of international business, you can't just rely on half a brain."[26]

Despite all our research into the brain in recent years, we are barely scratching the surface of how it works. What goes on inside a human head in this small mass of matter is so complex, how can anyone not be filled with awe?

When we encounter the complexity of the brain, a variety of questions press upon us, not the least of which is how such a delicate instrument came into being. What is it about the nature of the universe that, from the Big Bang billions of years ago, a vast array of galaxies sprang into being, giving rise to a planet on which exist creatures with the capacity for conscious exploration of what we call the creation. In other words, how did the universe ever birth an instrument so complex that it enables the universe to be conscious of itself?

As fascinating as the question of origins is, there is another question that some of us ask when we behold the wonder of the human brain. We want to know what the brain is capable of. What is our potential?

As we survey the myriad forms that comprise the world around us, once we balance our brain, what are we capable of doing with these forms? What's the potential of the creation in the hands of a balanced brain?

So far, we are only catching glimpses of something glorious, like trekking to the top of a mountain and seeing the vast array of creation that's before us, then realizing how much there is yet to explore.

Though I find the question of "how" the universe gave birth to consciousness fascinating, I am even more intrigued by the "what" question. In other words, I am more of an applications engineer. I want to know how we can apply our consciousness to the development and beneficial use of the creation that gave rise to us.

When an applications engineer sees patterns in the created order, such a person seeks to understand the ramifications of the different patterns. What are the advantages of one type of pattern over another? How can we use these patterns to develop more useful applications?

For instance, a man planned to commit suicide. People who commit suicide don't really want to die, they just want to escape the pain they are experiencing. What they are seeking is peace. On the day this man had intended to end his life, he decided to try brain training. I wanted to know what he was thinking as he left his first training sessions that day. I wasn't so much interested in how his brain was working, since I already measured his brain patterns, but in what he was thinking about. In other words, I wasn't concerned with analyzing him but in the tangible results of balancing his brain.

As it turned out, he was thinking about what he would fix for dinner that evening! His thoughts were also on what was going on in the lives of those close to him, as well as on the tasks he needed to accomplish to get his life moving forward again.

How wonderful that this man, who had planned to be dead by the end of the day, was thinking about an entirely different array of issues than where and how he would commit suicide and whether he had left appropriate instructions in the note he had written for his family! Instead of focusing on ending his life, his mind was engaging life in a meaningful way.

When we balance the brain, our mental content changes. Instead of our thoughts closing in on us, our mind begins expanding toward an infinite horizon.

You Can Take Charge of Your Life

There are elements of life over which we seemingly have no control. For instance, if you are tall and have blue eyes, you had nothing to do with it. Your genetics are a given.

We also have little control over certain elements of our environment. If you are driving down the street and a vehicle runs a red light and collides with you, it's an event that's outside your control.

Despite that we can do nothing to change some aspects of our life, our neural network is our entry into every area of life, including those areas we can't control. It affects our physiology, our thinking, our emotions, our creativity, our ability to learn, the values we hold, the spiritual path we follow, and even the hobbies we enjoy. Though we can't alter those things in life that are a given, what we make of our life in the face of them is greatly determined by our brain patterns.

A balanced brain and an unbalanced brain experience these realities in fundamentally different ways.

If your brain causes you to tighten and stay tightened in response to something in your environment, you'll use up a lot of energy. In due course, physiologically and psychologically, you'll start breaking down.

On the other hand, if your brain exhibits greater flexibility, you are more likely to go through a trauma and come out the other side without retaining long-term tightness and tension. In other words, whatever situation we find ourselves in, a brain that's balanced has more flexibility, more elasticity, so our functioning isn't so easily disrupted on a permanent basis.

Brain training seeks to impart the ability to respond in a fitting manner to whatever our situation may be and whatever may befall us. When we are in homeostasis, we heal better, perform tasks better, feel better, think better, and tend to excel in all the areas of life in which we wish to express ourselves.

Contentment coupled with optimum performance is a fine goal for all of us.

With an optimized brain, we make better partners, better parents, and become better people in the world. We take greater responsibility for our life.

We can see this readily from sports, where the ability to excel when our brain is balanced is evident. A person with a balanced brain has more accurate timing, increased strength, and improved agility—something that can be demonstrated by anyone on the golf course or with a set of barbells. Whether a person is a batter in a baseball game, a wide receiver or quarterback on a football field, a shooter or a defensive player in a basketball tournament, a swimmer in a race, or a dancer in a competition, a balanced brain can make all the difference by helping them pick up that split-second advantage. The difference between winners and losers in most Olympic contests has been less than a second.

A swimmer who had been swimming competitively for fifteen years trained her brain. She finished training on a Friday, competed on Saturday, and broke her twenty-year record that day. She was a sprinter. When she hit the water, she realized she hit it way before anybody else. She had an edge. That's all we need to excel in any area of life—just an edge.

When we relax the back of our tongue, we develop a dominant alpha brainwave pattern in certain parts of our brain. If you watch a film of Michael Jordan running down the basketball court on a fast break, where he's basically all alone, he is *in the zone,* at least in this aspect of his life. His tongue is flopping back and forth in his mouth, literally hanging out. Jordan was so incredible on the court because when he approached the basket on a fast break and faced a defender, he had the ability to move around the defender and to the basket like lightening. His tongue went into his mouth like a lizard, his jaw locked, and his legs exploded into action. As he leapt into the air, it was as if he could suspend himself there. Jordan had a huge natural energy reserve he could release when it was needed the most. It's not just that he was born this way. Peak performance isn't just about having a reservoir of capability, it's being able to apply this capability. Jordan was as great as he was at basketball because he could control his energy.

After training their brain, it's not just in the arena that someone in athletics tends to excel. Their success in competition is reflected in their personal life. Sadly, we often hear stories of athletes who abuse drugs, get into fights, or even beat their spouse. How can someone society holds up as a hero, who enjoys not only fame but also a fortune that allows them to lead a luxurious lifestyle, stray so far from a wholesome state of mind that they digress into drugs or family violence? If you were to see a brain assessment of such individuals, you would understand why. The person isn't being guided by their logical mind but by an unbalanced brain pattern. Athletes who train their brain not only reap the benefits in their performance, but also in their character.

Brain training not only puts people in the zone but also empowers them to become better human beings. Consider the case of an eleven-year-old golfer who was already exceptional and expected to go professional. His parents were concerned because he wasn't doing well academically or socially among his peers, so they wanted him to train his brain. At the same time, they were worried that if training increased his academic and social skills, his golf game might deteriorate. Training doesn't lower potential. The young man started doing well in school, and his friendships and ability to get along at home greatly improved. He also soared to a high national ranking in his golf game.

In training the brain, the aim isn't to alter a particular pattern for a specific purpose. For instance, there's no particular pattern so a person can sleep better, or one to become free of depression, or to rid us of a specific disease, or even to achieve a new level of creativity such as improving our artistic ability or our game of golf.

The only agenda in brain training is to help the brain become balanced and in harmony. When the playing field is level, the individual will in due course be able to accomplish what they want and need to accomplish.

In the Zone

As a quite different example of how a person begins to unleash their potential once they begin to see themselves and awaken to their own inner being, I have in my office a painting of a dancer by an artist who for twenty-three years painted still life, primarily pots and flowers. The name of the painting is significant: *In the Zone.*

This artist went through a course of brain training, which enabled her to see her artistic talent in a new light. She realized that, all her life, she had acted out an image of herself bequeathed to her by her parents, who had wanted her to paint pots and flowers because they believed this was what she would be best at painting. Because she relied on a borrowed sense of herself that was a reflection of her parents, what they thought she should paint is what she had painted ever since she took up art as a career—and she indeed painted the pots and flowers well, as her parents predicted.

By training her brain, this artist caught a glimpse of her *own* artistic passion—of an aspect of life for which she really had a *feel.* Once she recognized what her real passion was, she painted *In the Zone.* She has gone on to be more of a modern impressionistic painter of dancers who express through their dancing what it is to be in the zone.

When this artist became attuned to her own feelings instead of following the concept ingrained in her by her parents, her artwork came alive in a whole new dimension. Beneath the static and controlled still-life paintings she created for over twenty years lay a jewel, and all she needed was a channel to access it. She couldn't get to it by herself. She couldn't get to it by seeing herself in the mirror of her parents. She even had seen a tremendous number of impressionistic paintings in her life, but they couldn't awaken her own essence as an artist because that particular neural highway wasn't yet open.

Our Human Potential Unfolds

The brain's ability to observe itself is the key to the world's transformation into a peaceful and loving planet. When people begin to view the world through the lens of love rather than fear, the world itself becomes a better place. An optimized brain begins to see the potential for an optimized world. Humanity begins to reach for its limitless potential.

We asked in the Introduction: What could we do with the mind were our brain truly its faithful servant? What might we become aware of if our brain were finely tuned?

In an experiment to understand the capabilities of the human brain, a man climbs aboard a helicopter in the city of Rome in Italy. He has never seen the city before, and he is blindfolded so that he cannot catch even a glimpse of his surroundings until the moment the blindfold is removed. There is a camera on top of his head, which allows those conducting the experiment to record exactly what the man sees.

The helicopter tours the man over the city of Rome for three and a half hours, until the entire city has been systematically traversed.

After the helicopter lands, the man is taken into a room where a spread of thirty-five feet of white drawing paper is attached to a wall. There, with pencils, the man will draw what he saw from the helicopter.

The artist's rendition of the city of Rome is stunningly accurate, even though he has never seen any of it before. He draws every roofline, every window, every car, and every bus on the streets of the city—and he draws them to scale. It takes him three days to accomplish this.

The artist has been diagnosed with Autistic Spectrum Disorder (ASD), and he is a living demonstration of the incredible power of the brain—a power that few of us tap into very successfully in our everyday lives.

What possibilities exist in the brain? Most of us have an extremely limited view of our capabilities, yet our potential is beyond anything we have imagined. We all have the potential for greatness in us. Brain training can help release it. As our technology improves, the release of potential for specific individuals will generate release of even greater potential for whole communities, and eventually for entire nations and our world as a whole.

Our future is infinite, and all of this infinite potential exists today in the *limitless you*, waiting to be unleashed.

Bibliography

Aamodt, Sandra, PhD; Wang, Sam, PhD. 2008. *Welcome to Your Brain: Why You Lose Your Car Keys but Never Forget How to Drive and Other Puzzles of Everyday Life.* New York: Bloomsbury.

Begley, Sharon. 2007. *Train Your Mind, Change Your Brain.* New York: Ballantine Books.

Braden, Gregg. 2008. *The Spontaneous Healing of Belief.* Carlsbad, CA: Hay House.

Breggin, Peter R., MD. 2008. *Medication Madness: A Psychiatrist Exposes the Dangers of Mood-Altering Drugs.* New York: St. Martin's Press.

Carter, Rita. 1998. *Mapping the Mind.* Berkeley and Los Angeles, CA: University of California Press.

Doidge, Norman, MD. 2007. *The Brain That Changes Itself: Stories of Personal Triumph from Frontiers of Brain Science.* New York: Penguin.

Edelman, Gerald M., MD, PhD. 2006. *Second Nature.* New Haven, CT: Yale University Press.

Fehmi, Les, PhD; Robbins, Jim. 2007. *The Open-Focus Brain: Harnessing the Power of Attention to Heal Mind and Body.* Boston, MA: Trumpeter Books/ Shambhala.

Montague, Read. 2006. *Why Choose This Book?* New York: Dutton.

Restak, Richard, MD. 2006. *The Naked Brain.* New York: Three Rivers Press.

Schwartz, Jeffrey M, MD; Begley, Sharon. 2002. *The Mind & the Brain: Neuroplasticity and the Power of Mental Force.* New York: Regan Books.

Tiller, William, PhD. 1997. *Science and Human Transformation: Subtle Energies, Intentionality and Consciousness.* Walnut Creek, CA: Pavior.

Tiller, William, PhD; Dibble, Jr., Walter E., PhD; Kohane, Michael J., PhD. 2001. *Conscious Acts of Creation: The Emergence of a New Physics.* Walnut Creek, CA: Pavior.

Endnotes

1. You can see the algorithm in action on websites such as movielens.org, provided by the University of Minnesota. The service is free and they have a library of tens of thousands of movies and over 700,000 movie views. You choose movies you've seen, rate how you liked them, and the algorithms pick other movies you are likely to enjoy. If other members of your family or your friends also select movies, you can develop a library of recommendations for each and also discover what movies you would enjoy viewing together.

I had studied data from the University of Minnesota research on twins, which showed that people make choices based on their genetic makeup and not merely in response to their biographical data or socioeconomic status. For instance, if two twins are separated and one enters a high economic bracket while the other is in a low bracket, if the one in the high bracket buys a Maserati, the twin who can't afford such a luxury vehicle likely shares the same appreciation for the Maserati and has a picture of one on their desk. As a result of the development of this preference-matching algorithm, I was asked to appear on ABC News Nightline, which featured our work in a half-hour special called Soul Mates.

2. Anon. Mental health in the United States. Prevalence of diagnosis and medication treatment for attention-deficit/hyperactivity disorder–United States, 2003. Morb Mortal Wkly Rep 54:842–847, 2005.

National Institute of Mental Health (2003). Attention Deficit Hyperactivity Disorder (NIH Publication No. 03-3572). Available online: http://www.nimh.nih.gov/publicat/adhd.cfm.

Pritchard, D. "Attention deficit hyperactivity disorder in children." Clinical Evidence 2006 June (15): 331-344 (PMID: 16973014).

Kessler, R.C.; Adler, L.; Barkley, R.; et al. "The prevalence and correlates of adult ADHD in the United States: results from the National Comorbidity Survey Replication." American Journal of Psychiatry 163:716–723, 2006.

Faraone, S.V.; Biederman, J. "Prevalence of adult ADHD in the United States." Paper presented at the American Psychiatric Association annual meeting, New York, 2008.

3. With so many children now taking psychiatric drugs, Dr. Peter Breggin believes it is no exaggeration to say that we are damaging the brains and suppressing the mental function of millions of our children. For the most up-to-date information about the over-medication of children and the over-diagnosing of children with psychiatric disorders see:

Breggin, Peter R., MD. *Brain-Disabling Treatments in Psychiatry.* 2008. New York: Springer Publishing Co.

Svetlov, S.I.; Kobeissy, F.H.; and Gold, M.S. "Performance enhancing, non-prescription use of Ritalin: a comparison with amphetamines and cocaine." Journal of Addictive Disorders 26 (4): 1-6 (2007).

Wilens, T.E.; et al. "Does stimulant therapy of attention-deficit/hyperactivity disorder beget substance abuse: A meta analysis review of the literature." Pediatrics 111 (1): 179-185 (2003).

4. Norretranders, Tor. 1988. *The User Illusion: Cutting Consciousness Down to Size.* New York: Viking.

5. For people unfamiliar with emails, the process is rather like flushing liquid through a network of pipes. In order to make the best use of the pipes, several different types of liquids are all sent through the pipes at the same time. Each liquid has a distinct color and consistency, yet they are completely intermingled as they flow through the pipes. Blue and yellow might mix to make the liquid appear green, but at the other end of the pipe they are separated out into their original colors again. Even though the different colors and consistencies intermingle, blended together as if they were all one, at the end of the process—once the turbulence that mixes them stops—they separate out just as easily as oil and water.

6. The New England Journal of Medicine reported that in published trials, about sixty percent of people taking antidepressants report significant relief from depression, compared with forty percent of those taking placebos. However, when unpublished trials were included, antidepressants outperform placebos by only a small margin. The New England Journal of Medicine, Volume 358:252-260, January 17, 2009, No. 3.

"... according to testimony given in the fall of 2004 to the Congressional Energy and Commerce Committee, about half of all studies of anti-depressants have not shown in adults that the SSRI drugs are significantly more effective than a placebo alone. Even worse, insignificant results were found in two thirds of the studies in which children were given anti-depressants and compared to children given a placebo. This is not well understood by the general public. Please note that these research findings certainly do not prove that anti-depressants are entirely ineffective (in fact, half the studies may suggest anti-depressants yield some benefits), but these results cast considerable doubt on the effectiveness of the drugs. Psychiatrists know the effectiveness of anti-depressants is limited; they commonly point out that anti-depressants do not help about ⅓ of their depressed patients." Psych Central: The Use of Anti-Depressants, Clay Tucker-Ladd, PhD.

7. "But the body adapts to this 'intrusive' addition to what is a very complex and delicately balanced system and so the medication becomes less effective. This accounts for why so many people on antidepressants often have to increase dosages, change types of medication, etc." www.clinicaldepression. co.uk/Treating_Depression/controlling.html.

8. Peter R. Breggin, MD, argues that many categories of psychiatric drugs can cause potentially horrendous reactions. Prozac, Paxil, Zoloft, Adderall, Ritalin, Concerta, Xanax, lithium, Zyprexa, and other psychiatric medications may spellbind patients into believing they are improved when too often they are becoming worse. Psychiatric drugs drive some people into psychosis, mania, depression, suicide, agitation, compulsive violence and loss of self-control without the individuals realizing that their medications have deformed their way of thinking and feeling. Breggin, Peter R., MD. 2008. *Medication Madness: A Psychiatrist Exposes the Dangers of Mind-altering Medications*. New York: St. Martin's Press.

9. "In thousands of research studies, the treatment of depression with anti-depressants alone has been found to produce the highest rate of relapse, compared to what are considered effective therapies in the treatment of depression." www.clinicaldepression.co.uk/Treating_Depression/controlling.html.

10. The Washington Post, Thursday, Dec. 14, 2006.

"Antidepressants increase the risk compared to placebo of suicidal thinking and behavior (suicidality) in children, adolescents, and young adults in short-term studies of major depressive disorder (MDD) and other psychiatric disorders." Revisions to Product Labeling: www.fda.gov/CDER/DRUG/antidepressants/antidepressants_label_change_2007.pdf.

11. "Relapse rates for addictive diseases usually are in the range of 50% to 90%." Relapse rates for addiction range from 40% to 60%. "Alcohol/drug addiction is a chronic relapsing disorder." Caron: Comprehensive Addiction Treatment. www.caron.org/current-statistics.

12. "These findings suggest that, compared with placebo, the new-generation antidepressants do not produce clinically significant improvements in depression in patients who initially have moderate or even very severe depression, but show significant effects only in the most severely depressed patients. The findings also show that the effect for these patients seems to be due to decreased responsiveness to placebo, rather than increased responsiveness to medication. Given these results, the researchers conclude that there is little reason to prescribe new-generation antidepressant medications to any but the most severely depressed patients unless alternative treatments have been ineffective." Initial Severity and Antidepressant Benefits: A Meta-Analysis of Data Submitted to the Food and Drug Administration. PLOS Medicine, a peer-reviewed open-access journal published by the Public Library of Science.

13. "Acute response to antidepressant treatment is not always sustained. Loss of effect of antidepressant therapy appears to occur with most or all antidepressants." Oluboka, Oloruntoba Jacob, MB, BS, Halifax, NS; Persad, Emmanuel, MB, BS, London, Ontario: HealthyPlace.com Depression Community.

14. "After demonstrating that 30 minutes of brisk exercise three times a week is just as effective as drug therapy in relieving the symptoms of major depression in the short term, medical center researchers have now shown that continued exercise greatly reduces the chances of the depression returning. The new study, which followed the same participants for an additional six months, found that patients who continued to exercise after completing the initial trial were much less likely to see their depression return than the other patients. Only 8 percent of patients in the exercise group had their depression return, while

38 percent of the drug-only group and 31 percent of the exercise-plus-drug group relapsed. The research was supported by grants from the National Institutes of Health (NIH)." Study: Exercise Has Long-Lasting Effect on Depression, September 22, 2000, Duke University Office of News & Communications.

15. Treatment-Emergent Adverse Experience Incidence in Placebo-Controlled Clinical Trials (Percent of Patients Reporting)

Adverse Experience WELLBUTRIN Patients
(n = 323) Placebo Patients
(n = 185)

The first figure listed is the percentage of people in the study, and the next is the percentage of people in the placebo group who experienced adverse effects.

Cardiovascular

Cardiac arrhythmias	5.3	4.3%
Dizziness	22.3	16.2
Hypertension	4.3	1.6
Hypotension	2.5	2.2
Palpitations	3.7	2.2
Syncope	1.2	0.5
Tachycardia	10.8	8.6

Dermatologic

Pruritus	2.2	0.0
Rash	8.0	6.5

Gastrointestinal

Anorexia	18.3	18.4
Appetite increase	3.7	2.2
Constipation	26.0	17.3
Diarrhea	6.8	8.6
Dyspepsia	3.1	2.2
Nausea/vomiting	22.9	18.9
Weight gain	13.6	22.7
Weight loss	23.2	23.2

Genitourinary

Impotence	3.4	3.1%
Menstrual complaints	4.7	1.1
Urinary frequency	2.5	2.2
Urinary retention	1.9	2.2

Musculoskeletal

Arthritis	3.1	2.7

Neurological

Akathisia	1.5	1.1
Akinesia/bradykinesia	8.0	8.6
Cutaneous temperature disturbance	1.9	1.6
Dry mouth	27.6	18.4
Excessive sweating	22.3	14.6
Headache/migraine	25.7	22.2
Impaired sleep quality	4.0	1.6
Increased salivary flow	3.4	3.8
Insomnia	18.6	15.7
Muscle spasms	1.9	3.2
Pseudoparkinsonism	1.5	1.6
Sedation	19.8	19.5
Sensory disturbance	4.0	3.2
Tremor	21.1	7.6

Neuropsychiatric

Agitation	31.9	22.2
Anxiety	3.1	1.1
Confusion	8.4	4.9
Decreased libido	3.1	1.6
Delusions	1.2	1.1
Disturbed concentration	3.1	3.8
Euphoria	1.2	0.5
Hostility	5.6	3.8

Nonspecific

Fatigue	5.0	8.6

Fever/chills	1.2	0.5%

Respiratory
Upper respiratory complaints	5.0	11.4

Special Senses
Auditory disturbance	5.3	3.2
Blurred vision	14.6	10.3
Gustatory disturbance	3.1	1.1

16. http://www.nlm.nih.gov/medlineplus/druginfo/medmaster/a695033. html.

Rappley, MD. "Clinical practice: Attention deficit hyperactivity disorder." New England Journal of Medicine 352 92): 165-173 (2005).

17. Jelinek, Pauline: Associated Press, April 18, 2008.

18. 10th Special Report to the U.S. Congress on Alcohol and Health, June 2000, U.S. Department of Health and Human Services.

19. The National Institute of Drug Abuse says that "treatment of addiction is as successful as treatment of other chronic diseases, such as diabetes, hypertension, and asthma." But this isn't very successful. We estimate that about 12% of those beginning Twelve Step programs are successful two or more years later. Also, A. Orange writes that "rarely have we seen a person fail who has thoroughly followed our path. Those who do not recover are those who cannot or will not give themselves completely to this simple program, usually men and women who are constitutionally incapable of being honest with themselves. There are such unfortunates. They are not at fault; they seem to have been born that way." A.A. Big Book, 3rd & 4th Editions, William G. Wilson, page 58. Nothing could be further from the truth. The success rate for A.A. and N.A. depends on who is doing the counting, how they are counting, and what they are counting or measuring. A 5% success rate is nothing more than the rate of spontaneous remission in alcoholics and drug addicts. That is, out of any given group of alcoholics or drug addicts, approximately 5% per year will just wise up, and quit killing themselves. They just get sick and tired of being sick and tired, and of watching their friends die. (And something between 1% and 3% of their friends

do die annually, so that is a big incentive.) They often quit with little or no official treatment or help. Some actually detox themselves on their own couches, or in their own beds, or locked in their own closets. Often, they don't go to a lot of meetings. They just quit, all on their own, or with the help of a couple of good friends who keep them locked up for a few days while they go through withdrawal. A.A. and N.A. true believers insist that addicts can't successfully quit that way, but they do, every day.

I agree with R. G. Smart, who calculated a spontaneous remission rate for alcoholism of between 3.7 and 7.4 percent per year. As a simple rule of thumb, the middle value of 5 or 5.5 percent per year is quite believable.

20. A comparison of transurethral resection of the prostate and biopsy detection among more than 18,000 men with normal prostate-specific antigen (PSA) levels and digital rectal exam (DRE) results—"a low-risk group"—showed that 25% of that population had prostate cancer. New England Journal of Medicine, 2003; 349:213-22.

21. "12.03% of women born today will be diagnosed with cancer of the breast at some time during their lifetime. This number can also be expressed as 1 in 8 women will be diagnosed with cancer of the breast during their lifetime." National Cancer Institute: Surveillance Epidemiology and End Results. http://seer.cancer.gov/statfacts/html/breast.html

22. Mattes, Aaron: www.stretchingusa.com. Aaron explained in a personal communication: "The stretch is held less than two seconds with the agonist contracting for less than one pound of assistive pressure. Over two seconds aggravates the stretch reflex and becomes isometric resistance, which results in less blood flow and oxygen; and with trauma, spinal cord, neurological problems, etc., the results are monumental. The best athletes in the world are also using it successfully."

23. World Health Organization. Global burden of neurological disorders and mental health (2005).
Science, April 2002. http://www.sciencemag.org

24. Hazlett, Dr. Heather Cody: University of North Carolina at Chapel Hill, University of North Carolina News Services, December 5, 2005, No. 608.

25. Professor Simon Baron-Cohen, of Cambridge University, speaking at the British Association Festival of Science in York, September 11, 2007, presented research to indicate that fetal testosterone is correlated with autistic traits. His research involved 235 children born in 1999 whose levels of testosterone experienced in the womb had been measured, and who, while not themselves autistic, manifest autistic-like traits. "Children with autism seem to have a very strong exaggeration of the male profile," Baron-Cohen concluded, adding, "They have a strong interest in systems, and difficulty empathizing." A study of 90,000 samples from Denmark's Biobank, gathered from amniocentesis, is now underway.

26. Rae-Dupree, Janet: "Da Vinci, Retrofitted for the Modern Age," The New York Times, June 1, 2008.

If you like this book, you may also want to investigate these transformational books by Namaste Publishing:

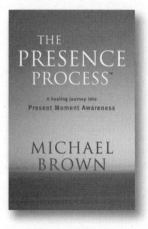

The Presence Process
MICHAEL BROWN

Until 1989, South African-born Michael Brown was living what he called a blissfully unconscious life as a music journalist. He then developed an acutely painful neurological condition for which conventional medicine had neither cure nor relief. This caused him to set out on what became a nine-year odyssey of self-healing.

In showing us how to step beyond our personal physical, mental, and emotional afflictions and addictions, and by empowering us to facilitate ourselves into wholeness, The Presence Process takes a bold step into a new paradigm of healthcare.

The lucid flow of this text magnetically and gently draws us into a transformational experience that automatically grounds us into the vibrant radiance of present moment awareness, where we find our liberation, our healing, our innate wisdom.

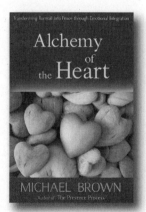

Alchemy of the Heart
Transforming Turmoil into Peace
Through Emotional Integration
MICHAEL BROWN

The causal point of the things that occur in our everyday experience isn't outside of us in the actions of others, but within each of us. During our early years, we are imprinted by the emotional condition of those responsible for us.

In *Alchemy of the Heart*, we are asked to become conscious of the ways we were imprinted and how these imprints drive our behavior. Our guide in achieving this course correction is the heart. The heart is our bridge to the vibrational dimension of reality, which is experienced as consciousness. The language of the heart is felt-perception. This alone can steer us in the right direction. It is not the same as our emotions, which have been distorted by our early years. Through felt-perception, the heart enables us to re-parent ourselves. Our own wholeness then meets our needs, not other people. This frees us to love unconditionally.

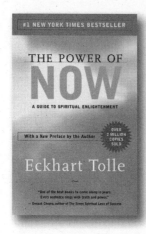

The Power of Now
A Guide to Spiritual Enlightenment
ECKHART TOLLE

Renowned spiritual teacher Eckhart Tolle takes us out of our analytical thoughts and reactive emotions, into the power that resides in the present moment. To offer no resistance to life is to be in a state of grace, ease, and lightness. This state is then no longer dependent upon things being in a certain way, good or bad. It seems almost paradoxical, yet when your inner dependency on form is gone, the general conditions of your life, the outer forms, tend to improve greatly. Things, people, or conditions that you thought you needed for your happiness now come to you with no struggle or effort on your part, and you are free to enjoy and appreciate them—while they last. All those things, of course, will still pass away, cycles will come and go, but with dependency gone there is no fear of loss anymore. Life flows with ease.

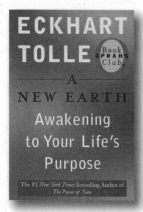

A New Earth
Awakening to Your Life's Purpose
ECKHART TOLLE

A New Earth presents readers with an honest look at the current state of humanity. Eckhart implores us to see and accept that this state, which is based on an erroneous identification with the egoic mind, is one of dangerous insanity. There is good news, however. There is an alternative to this potentially dire situation. Humanity now, perhaps more than in any previous time, has an opportunity to create a new, saner, more loving world. This will involve a radical inner leap from the current egoic consciousness to an entirely new one. In illuminating the nature of this shift in consciousness, Eckhart describes in detail how our current ego-based state of consciousness operates. Then gently, and in very practical terms, he leads us into this new consciousness. We will come to experience who we truly are—which is something infinitely greater than anything we currently think we are—and learn to live and breathe freely.

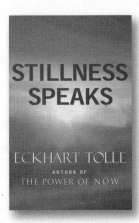

Stillness Speaks
ECKHART TOLLE

While spiritually profound, *Stillness Speaks* is also intensely practical. Eckhart tells us how to be with another in a relationship which can contain and weather all things, how to "sit" with a dying person, where to find wisdom, how to free ourselves of guilt, and how to control the runaway thinking mind. Underneath the words, between them, in the energy of presence conveyed by them, we find the power of stillness. This vibrantly alive state found only in the here and now is one with our Being and the field out of which everything arises.

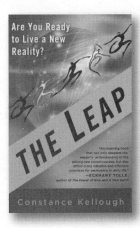

The Leap
Are You Ready to Live a New Reality?
CONSTANCE KELLOUGH,
Publisher of *The Power of Now*

The Leap is filled with hope for tomorrow. In our troubled world, it's easy to feel alone—and, in our era of campus shootings and terrorism, fearful. *The Leap* shows us that we are far from alone—that we are part of something so encompassing, we can never be alone. A global shift is occurring in which we are edging our way toward becoming one world. Now, we must link to a sense of inner connectedness that few experience yet on a daily basis, but that is essential if we are to interact with each other peacefully. As we become conscious of our inner oneness, we begin living from a different mindset. We experience a deep stillness, from which an intuitive wisdom arises to guide every aspect of our personal lives and how we respond to each other. *The Leap* not only changes how we make decisions as individuals, but also as leaders of organizations and countries. It provides the key to personal fulfillment—and the hope of the world.

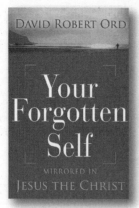

Your Forgotten Self
Mirrored in Jesus the Christ
DAVID ROBERT ORD

If you are like millions of others who seek to understand Jesus, and perhaps hope someday to be like him, chances are you don't experience the "peace that passes understanding" and "joy unspeakable" that his first disciples did. The reason is simple—you think of Jesus as *different* from yourself. In the view of Jesus' early followers, we have no hope of enjoying the fulfilling life Jesus lived as long as we regard him as essentially different from us. To Peter, John, Mary, and Paul, Jesus was the embodiment of our true nature—a reflection of who we really are. *Your Forgotten Self* invites you to experience yourself through new eyes. To be a believer is to see yourself mirrored in Jesus. To have faith is to understand yourself as Jesus understood himself. When this happens, the power of the Christ floods your everyday life. You begin to live as Jesus in the present moment.

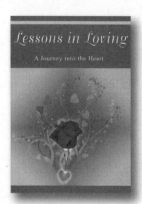

Lessons in Loving
A Journey into the Heart
DAVID ROBERT ORD

(audio book)

We seek fulfillment in relationships, not realizing that our greatest desire is to be *ourselves* in the fullest sense. For only when we can truly be who *we* really are is the heart-to-heart connection for which we long possible. Once you connect with your own essence, instead of romance fading as the years go by, you find it increasing. Instead of passion waning, it grows stronger. True to *yourself* at last, you experience the fascination, sense of wonder, and excitement of being with another. If the bottom has fallen out of your life, you'll especially find this book helpful. What do you do when the pain of loss is so great that you don't know what to do with yourself? How do you cope with the overwhelming sadness, the incredible loneliness? Anyone going through a devastating disappointment, such as divorce or loss of a loved one, needs the insight that's in this book. Join David Ord on a journey of self-discovery, and learn the pathway to deeply fulfilling relationships.

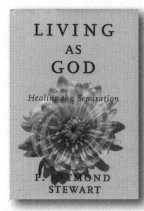

Living As God
Healing the Separation
P. RAYMOND STEWART

We may have for a long time been under the impression that our individual and collective spiritual awakening is a journey that we must make *towards* God. This is a perception born of the consciousness of separation. The presence of a book such as *Living as God* is proof that our growing awareness of our Divinity is actually a tidal wave of remembrance that is crashing down onto our seemingly beached humanity. P. Raymond Stewart communicates with effortless simplicity that it is through the acknowledgement of our shared inner Presence that we shall awaken to the realization that we are already submerged and saturated in God. Each page of *Living as God* soaks our awareness in the dawning realization that God is already present as us. Right here, right now.

Additional books, CDs, and DVDs by
Namaste Publishing authors may be found at:
www.namastepublishing.com

NAMASTE PUBLISHING

P.O. Box 62084, Vancouver, British Columbia, Canada V6J 4A3
www.namastepublishing.com

Our Publishing Mission is to make available healing and transformational publications
that acknowledge, celebrate, and encourage our readers to live
from their divine essence and thereby come to remember who they really are.

———

If you liked this book, you may also want to become aware of our
other transformational publications, including cds and dvds
exclusive to Namaste Publishing's website.
To do this, please visit our website at:

www.namastepublishing.com

———

To receive full benefit from our books, we invite you to read our daily blog:

The Compassionate Eye

———

We also invite you to sign up for our free monthly Newsletter in which
we bring you articles by our staff writers, book and movie reviews,
frequent downloads from our authors, and information on
Namaste Publishing's forthcoming publications.

———

If you want to place an order for any of our publications, find out
the teaching schedules of our authors, schedule one of our authors
for a teaching or speaking event, or sign up for our BLOG and
NEWSLETTER, please visit our home page:

www.namastepublishing.com